Gastrointesti

Gastrointestinal Imaging Cases

Angela D. Levy, MD
Professor of Radiology
Department of Radiology
Georgetown University Hospital
Washington, DC

Koenraad J. Mortele, MD
Associate Professor of Radiology
Harvard Medical School
Beth Israel Deaconess Medical Center
Boston, Massachusetts

Benjamin M. Yeh, MD
Professor of Radiology
Department of Radiology and
Biomedical Imaging
University of California, San Francisco
San Francisco, California

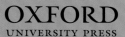

OXFORD
UNIVERSITY PRESS

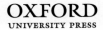

OXFORD
UNIVERSITY PRESS

Oxford University Press is a department of the University of Oxford.
It furthers the University's objective of excellence in research, scholarship,
and education by publishing worldwide.

Oxford   New York
Auckland   Cape Town   Dar es Salaam   Hong Kong   Karachi
Kuala Lumpur   Madrid   Melbourne   Mexico City   Nairobi
New Delhi   Shanghai   Taipei   Toronto

With offices in
Argentina   Austria   Brazil   Chile   Czech Republic   France   Greece
Guatemala   Hungary   Italy   Japan   Poland   Portugal   Singapore
South Korea   Switzerland   Thailand   Turkey   Ukraine   Vietnam

Oxford is a registered trademark of Oxford University Press in the UK
and certain other countries.

Published in the United States of America by
Oxford University Press
198 Madison Avenue, New York, NY 10016

Library of Congress Cataloging-in-Publication Data
Levy, Angela D.
Gastrointestinal imaging cases/Angela D. Levy, Koenraad Mortele, Benjamin M. Yeh.
    p.; cm. — (Cases in radiology)
Includes bibliographical references and indexes.
ISBN 978–0–19–975943–9 (alk. paper) — ISBN 978–0–19–998220–2 (alk. paper) —
ISBN 978–0–19–998221–9 (alk. paper)
I. Mortele, Koenraad J.   II. Yeh, Benjamin.   III. Title.   IV. Series: Cases in radiology.
[DNLM: 1. Digestive System Diseases—diagnosis—Case Reports.   2. Diagnostic Imaging—
Case Reports. WI 141]
616.3′075—dc23
2012034465

This material is not intended to be, and should not be considered, a substitute for medical or other professional
advice. Treatment for the conditions described in this material is highly dependent on the individual
circumstances. And while this material is designed to offer accurate information with respect to the subject
matter covered and to be current as of the time it was written, research and knowledge about medical and health
issues are constantly evolving and dose schedules for medications are being revised continually, with new side
effects recognized and accounted for regularly. Readers must therefore always check the product information
and clinical procedures with the most up-to-date published product information and data sheets provided by
the manufacturers and the most recent codes of conduct and safety regulation. The publisher and the authors
make no representations or warranties to readers, express or implied, as to the accuracy or completeness of this
material. Without limiting the foregoing, the publisher and the authors make no representations or warranties as
to the accuracy or efficacy of the drug dosages mentioned in the material. The authors and the publisher do not
accept, and expressly disclaim, any responsibility for any liability, loss or risk that may be claimed or incurred as a
consequence of the use and/or application of any of the contents of this material.

9 8 7 6 5 4 3 2 1
Printed in China
on acid-free paper

For my husband, Asa, and his loving support.

ADL

To Dejana, who teaches me everyday the essence of life with love, and my four
incredible children, Charlotte, Christophe, Mabel, and Mila.

KJM

To the low V/Q basketball team.

BMY

Preface

Modern gastrointestinal imaging integrates all currently existing imaging modalities including multi-detector row CT, MRI, ultrasound, scintigraphy, fluoroscopy, and radiography for the diagnosis and management of gastrointestinal diseases. These diseases occur in a wide range of organs in the abdomen and pelvis. They are encountered not only during the GI rotation, but also on virtually all rotations.

This casebook is a concise compilation of patients with classic gastrointestinal diseases evaluated by imaging. The practical teaching points in these cases are designed to be useful for practicing radiologists, radiology residents, medical students, and clinicians involved in the care of patients with gastrointestinal diseases.

For convenience, the cases are organized by organ. They are paginated for the reader to review the images as "unknown" followed by a discussion of the findings in the case, differential diagnosis, pertinent teaching points on the disease process, and management. The text is designed to highlight the most important features of each disease process that allow it to be diagnosed based on the images provided in the case.

This casebook is a companion and complement to our forthcoming Gastrointestinal Imaging textbook in the Oxford Rotations in Radiology Series.

The Publisher thanks the following for their time and advice:

Mark Anderson, University of Virginia
Sanjeev Bhalla, Mallinckrodt Institute of Radiology, Washington University
Michael Bruno, Penn State Hershey Medical Center
Melissa Rosado de Christenson, St. Luke's Hospital of Kansas City
Rihan Khan, University of Arizona
Angela Levy, Georgetown University
Alexander Mamourian, University of Pennsylvania
Stacy Smith, Brigham and Women's Hospital

Contents

Contributors

Michael A. Abramson, MD
Diagnostic Radiology Resident
Georgetown University Hospital
Washington, DC

Catherine Dewhurst, MD
Clinical Fellow Body MRI
Harvard Medical School
Beth Israel Deaconess Medical Center
Boston, MA

Garney Fendley, MD
San Francisco Veterans Affairs Medical
    Center
San Francisco, CA

Edward P. Harter, MD
Diagnostic Radiology Resident
Georgetown University Hospital
Washington, DC

Nasheen Hasan, DO, MPH
Assistant Professor of Clinical Radiology
Cornell Medical School
Lincoln Medical and Mental Health Center
Bronx, NY

Peter E. Humphrey, MD
Assistant Professor
University of New Mexico
School of Medicine
Albuquerque, NM

Taylor Jordan, MD
Clicnical Fellow
Abdominal Imaging Department of
    Radiology and Biomedical Imaging
University of California
San Francisco, CA

Marcia McCowin, MD
Clinical Professor of Radiology
University of California
San Francisco, CA

John Mongan, MD, PhD
Diagnostic Radiology Resident
Department of Radiology and Biomedical
    Imaging
University of California
San Francisco, CA

Jeff Mottola, MD
Attending Radiologist
Health Sciences Center
University of Mannitoba
Winnipeg, CA

Jennifer Nimhuircheartaigh, MD
Clinical Fellow Body MRI
Harvard Medical School
Beth Israel Deaconess Medical Center
Boston, MA

Bijal Patel, MD
Radiology Consultants Associated Calgary
Alberta Canada and Brigham and Women's
    Hospital Division of Abdominal
    Imaging and Intervention
Department of Radiology
Harvard Medical School
Boston, MA

Daniel A.T. Souza, MD
Clinical Fellow Brigham and Women's
    Hospital
Dana Farber Cancer Institute
Harvard Medical School
Boston, MA

Stefanie Weinstein, MD
San Francisco Veterans Affairs Medical
    Center
San Francisco, CA

Part 1   Pharynx and Esophagus

History

► 68-year-old man with dysphagia.

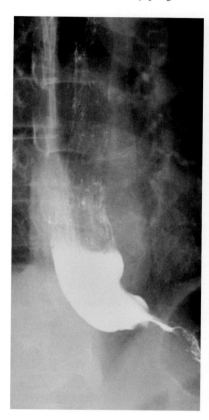 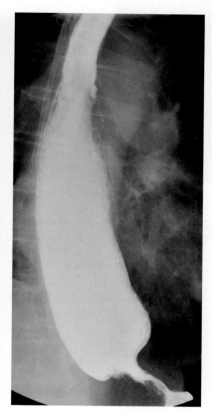

Case 1 Pseudoachalasia from an Adenocarcinoma of the Gastric Cardia

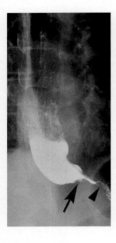 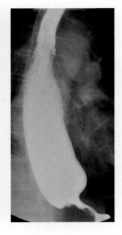

Findings

Esophagram shows a dilated esophagus with retained secretions. The distal esophagus tapers irregularly at the gastroesophageal junction. There is nodularity of the distal esophagus (left image, arrow) and in the region of the gastric cardia (left image, arrowhead).

Differential Diagnosis

- ▶ Primary achalasia: absence of primary peristalsis, smooth "beak-like" tapering of the distal esophagus. The degree of esophageal dilatation varies with the duration and severity of the disease.
- ▶ Scleroderma: dilated esophagus with a patulous gastroesophageal junction. If a peptic stricture is present, the appearance may be similar to achalasia.
- ▶ Peptic stricture: may cause proximal esophageal dilatation, but usually a hiatal hernia is present and aperistalsis is not a feature.
- ▶ Postoperative esophageal dilatation: aperistalsis, dilatation, and distal esophageal tapering may occur after a Nissen fundoplication. The fundoplication wrap is usually apparent.

Teaching Points

Pseudoachalasia, also called secondary achalasia, is narrowing of the distal esophagus from carcinoma of the gastroesophageal junction region or, rarely, from benign causes, such as Chagas disease. The radiographic presentation of pseudoachalasia is similar to primary achalasia because both conditions may produce a tapered narrowing of the distal esophagus, dilatation, and aperistalsis. Although pseudoachalasia may be indistinguishable from primary achalasia, features that suggest pseudoachalasia from carcinomas of the gastroesophageal region should always be sought out when interpreting barium studies. These include nodularity of the distal tapered segment, shouldering, or eccentricity from mass effect. The narrowed distal segment may be long, greater than 3.5 cm, in pseudoachalasia. Adenocarcinoma of the gastric cardia or distal esophagus are the most common malignancies seen with pseudoachalasia.

Management

Endoscopic visualization of the distal esophagus and gastric cardia with biopsy is necessary to establish the diagnosis.

Further Reading

1. Woodfield CA, Levine MS, Rubesin SE, Langlotz CP and Laufer I. Diagnosis of primary versus secondary achalasia: reassessment of clinical and radiographic criteria. *Am J Roentgenol.* 2000;*175*: 727–731.

History

► 90-year-old woman with non-cardiac, retrosternal chest pain. Barium esophagram is performed for evaluation.

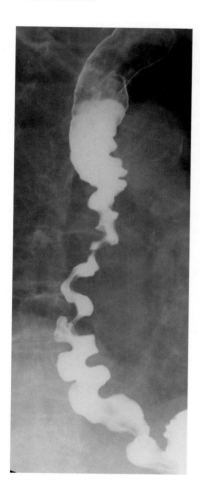

Case 2 Diffuse Esophageal Spasm

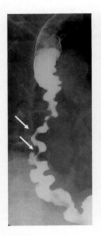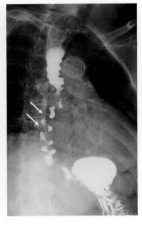

Findings

Spot (left) and overhead (right) images from barium esophagram show multiple, simultaneous, non-peristaltic esophageal contractions (long arrows), some of which efface the barium column.

Differential Diagnosis

▶ Nonspecific esophageal motility disorder: the preferred term for motility disorders (such as presbyesophagus) that show interrupted primary peristalsis and multiple, simultaneous, non-propulsive, low-amplitude esophageal contractions.

▶ Achalasia: characteristically atonic, dilated esophagus that lacks normal relaxation of the lower esophageal sphincter. The enlarged esophagus may take on a redundant "sigmoid" appearance that may resemble diffuse esophageal spasm (DES).

Teaching Points

DES is an infrequently encountered motility disorder of esophageal smooth muscle that usually affects the distal two-thirds of the esophagus. Patients may present with intermittent chest pain and/or dysphagia, which can vary in severity and duration. The dysphagia can be associated with ingestion of solids or liquids. Disorders of enteric motor innervation are believed to be responsible for the condition. Typically, the primary peristaltic wave is preserved in the cervical esophagus but becomes disrupted distally by the characteristic simultaneous high-pressure contractions that interrupt the barium column and impart the classic "corkscrew" appearance that may be seen on barium studies. Further evaluation may involve the documentation of high amplitude contractions with manometry in symptomatic patients.

Management

DES is a chronic condition that may or may not improve with therapy. If dietary modifications or a trial of proton pump inhibitors are unsuccessful, further medical management with long-acting nitrates, calcium channel blockers, botulinum injections may prove helpful. Surgical myotomy is reserved for patients who have failed medical management and is variably successful.

Further Readings

1. Grubel C, Borovicka J, Schwizer W, et al. Diffuse esophageal spasm. *Am J Gastroenterol.* 2008; *103*: 450–457.
2. Prabhakar A, Levine MS, Rubesin I, et al. Relationship between diffuse esophageal spasm and lower esophageal sphincter dysfunction on barium studies and manometry in 14 patients. *Am J Roentgenol.* 2004; *183*: 409–413.
3. Chen YM, Ott DJ, Hewson EG, et al. Diffuse esophageal spasm: radiographic and manometric correlation. *Radiology.* 1989; *170*(3): 807–810.

History

▶ 59-year-old woman with chronic dysphagia.

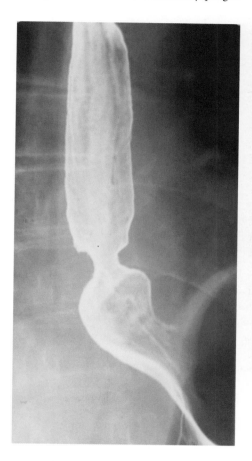 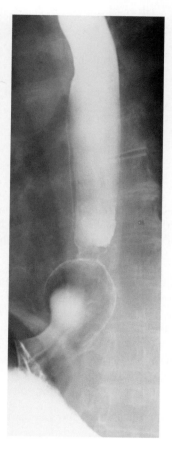

Case 3 Benign Distal Esophageal Stricture

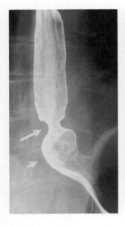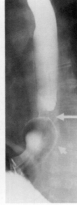

Findings

Spot images from a double-contrast barium esophagram show a fixed short segment of concentric luminal narrowing (long arrow) of the distal esophagus superior to a hiatal hernia (short arrow). The narrowed segment has smooth mucosal borders and obliquely angled shoulders relative to the normal lumen.

Differential Diagnosis

► Peristaltic contraction: would not manifest as a fixed segment of narrowing.
► Extrinsic compression: typically appears as eccentric rather than concentric narrowing.
► Achalasia: dilated proximal esophagus with tapered barium column at the gastroesophageal junction secondary to non-relaxation of the lower esophageal sphincter. A severe distal esophageal stricture could appear similar.
► Malignant stricture: irregularly marginated and may have associated mural nodularity, mucosal ulceration, or a mural mass.

Teaching Points

The majority of benign distal esophageal strictures are due to reflux esophagitis. On barium examination, these may appear as eccentric areas of luminal flattening or, if the scarring is severe or progressive, short segments of concentric fixed luminal narrowing. Concentric strictures are typically located just above a hiatal hernia, which occur from esophageal shortening secondary to the contraction produced by scar formation. Smooth mucosal margins and obliquely angled shoulders on barium examination imply benignity, and any irregularity should raise suspicion of a malignant cause. If superimposed columnar metaplasia (Barrett esophagus) is present along the strictured segment, the involved mucosa may exhibit a reticular appearance. Mucosal inflammation from medication tablets, Crohn disease, Behcet syndrome, and epidermolysis bullosa are other potential etiologies of benign distal esophageal strictures.

Management

For benign, symptomatic esophageal strictures from reflux esophagitis, non-surgical therapy with proton pump inhibitors is initiated. If symptoms persist, stricturoplasty with graded bougienage or balloon dilatation may be performed.

Further Readings

1. Levine MS, Rubesin SE. Diseases of the esophagus: diagnosis with esophagography. *RadioGraphics*. 2005; *237*(2): 414–427.
2. Lind CD. Dysphagia: evaluation and treatment. *Gastroenterol Clin N Am*. 2003; *32*: 553–575.
3. Gupta SS, Levine MS, Rubesin SE, et al. Usefulness of barium studies for differentiating benign and malignant strictures of the esophagus. *Am J Roentgenol*. 2003; *180*(3): 737–744.

History

▶ 62-year-old man with long history of alcoholism, recent 20-pound weight loss and two to three months of solid food dysphagia and odynophagia.

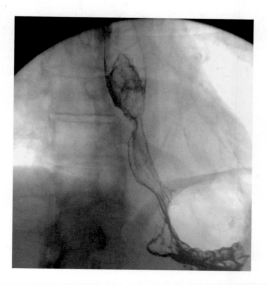

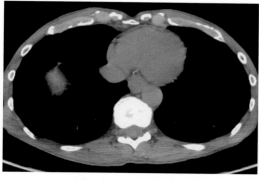

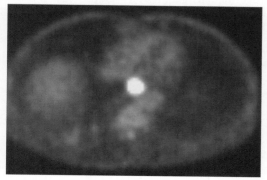

Case 4 Esophageal Cancer

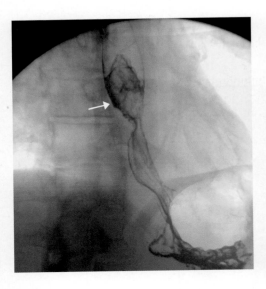
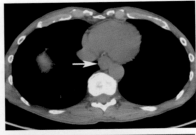
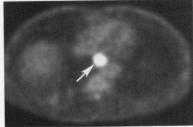

Findings

Esophagram (left) shows an irregular eccentric distal esophageal mass with shelf-like margins (arrow). CT image (top right) shows a thick-walled esophagus (arrow) with corresponding FDG avidity (arrow) on PET-CT image (bottom right). The fat plane between the mass and descending aorta is preserved.

Differential Diagnosis

► Barrett esophagus: short stricture with ulceration and a reticular mucosa at fluoroscopy. No associated mass.
► Extrinsic mass: lung cancer or mediastinal lymph nodes may compress and deviate the esophagus, causing smooth esophageal narrowing with obtuse angles.
► Esophageal varices: serpentine submucosal impressions in the esophagus that change in caliber with breathing, as opposed to tumors which remain fixed.

Teaching Points

Although esophageal cancer is relatively uncommon, it is the sixth leading cause of cancer deaths world-wide, and more than 50 percent of patients have unresectable tumors at the time of diagnosis. Cigarette smoking, male gender, substantial alcohol use, gastrointestinal reflux, obesity, and Barrett esophagus are predisposing factors, as are prior mediastinal radiation, achalasia, lye strictures and celiac disease. Esophagrams show esophageal cancer as a nodular mass with asymmetric irregular narrowing of the esophagus with shelf-like margins and ulcerations. In contrast, benign esophageal strictures tend to show smooth tapered symmetric narrowing. Early stage cancers are better detected and characterized with endoscopy. The incidence of adenocarcinoma has increased such that it is now similar to squamous cell carcinoma, possibly due to the increased incidence of reflux related Barrett esophagus. CT findings of advanced local spread include tumor infiltration of the peri-esophageal fat.

Management

Complete surgical resection results in a five-year survival rate of up to 80 percent, but higher stage tumors have a much poorer prognosis. Radiotherapy and chemotherapy are used for palliation.

Further Readings

1. Enzinger PC, Mayer RJ. Esophageal cancer. *N Engl J Med.* 2003; *349*: 22241–2252.
2. Lyer R, DuBrow R. Imaging of esophageal cancer. *Cancer Imaging.* 2004; *4*(2): 125–132.

History

▶ 30-year-old man with human immunodeficiency virus infection complains of severe odynophagia.

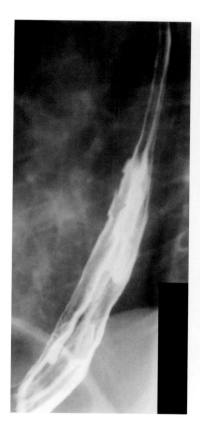
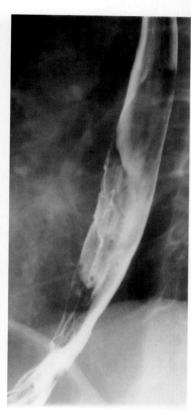

Case 5 CMV Esophagitis

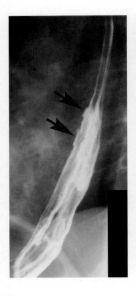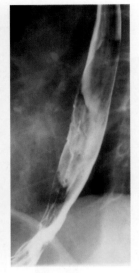

Findings

Double contrast esophagram shows two sharply marginated, shallow ulcers in the anterior distal esophagus (left image, arrows). The adjacent esophageal mucosa is normal.

Differential Diagnosis

▶ Herpes esophagitis: ulcers in herpes esophagitis are often indistinguishable from cytomegalovirus (CMV) ulcerations. However, giant ulcers (greater than 1 cm) usually do not occur in herpes esophagitis.
▶ Human immunodeficiency virus esophagitis: may produce giant ulcerations indistinguishable from CMV ulcers.

Teaching Points

CMV is a member of the herpes virus group. Clinically apparent infection occurs in immunosuppressed patients. CMV esophagitis is rare, primarily occurring in patients with acquired immunodeficiency syndrome (AIDS). Well defined esophageal ulcerations are the most common findings. The ulcerations are usually located in the mid or distal esophagus, resembling herpes virus ulcerations. On a double contrast barium esophagram, the ulcers are discrete with a radiolucent rim of surrounding edema. CMV may also produce giant ulcers that are greater than 1 cm.

Management

Endoscopic biopsy is necessary to distinguish between CMV, herpes, and HIV ulcerations.

Further Readings

1. Levine MS, Woldenberg, R, Herlinger H, Laufer, I . Opportunistic esophagitis in AIDS: radiographic diagnosis. *Radiology.* 1987; *165*: 815–820.
2. Teixidor HS, Honig CL, Norsoph E, et al. Cytomegalovirus infection of the alimentary canal: radiologic findings with pathologic correlation. *Radiology.* 1987; *163*: 317–323.

History

▸ 62-year-old man with dysphagia.

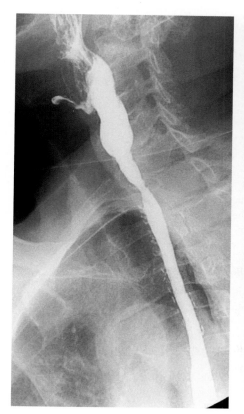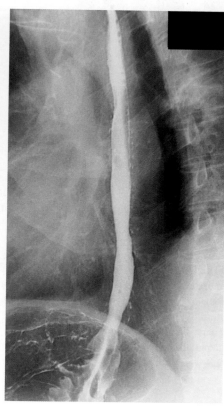

Case 6   Intramural Pseudodiverticulosis with Reflux Stricture

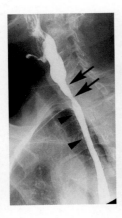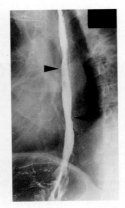

Findings

Esophagram shows a stricture (arrows) near the proximal esophageal sphincter. There are innumerable thin linear or flask-shaped outpouchings (arrowheads) throughout the thoracic esophagus.

Differential Diagnosis

▸ Esophagitis: ulcers in esophagitis communicate directly with the esophageal lumen. Intramural pseudodiverticula have a flask shape without apparent connection to the lumen.
▸ Perforation with extraluminal contrast extravasation: contrast flows away from the esophagus into the mediastinum or pleural space, and patients are usually symptomatic with pain, fever, or crepitus from a pneumomediastinum if present.
▸ Intramural esophageal dissection: associated with an injury to the esophagus. An intramural contrast channel typically parallels the wall of the esophagus producing a double barrel appearance, in contrast to pseudodiverticula, which are oriented perpendicular to the wall.

Teaching Points

Esophageal pseudodiverticulosis is an uncommon finding in the esophagus that occurs when oral contrast fills dilated ducts of deep mucous glands, which communicate with the esophageal lumen. Pseudodiverticulosis may be focal or may involve the esophagus diffusely. Although the etiology of the glandular duct dilatation and pseudodiverticulosis is not known, it is presumed to be related to chronic gastroesophageal reflux. Ninety percent of patients have an associated esophageal stricture. The stricture is commonly proximal to the pseudodiverticulosis. Most patients complain of dysphagia, which is related to the presence of the stricture. Esophageal carcinoma has been reported to occur with increased prevalence in patients with esophageal pseudodiverticulosis.

Management

The esophageal strictures associated with pseudodiverticulosis are responsible for the patient's symptoms and respond well to mechanical dilatation.

Further Readings

1. Levine MS, Moolten DN, Herlinger H, Laufer I. Esophageal intramural pseudodiverticulosis: a reevaluation. *Am J Roentgenol.* 1986; *147*(6): 1165–1170.
2. Plavsic BM, Chen MY, Gelfand DW, et al. Intramural pseudodiverticulosis of the esophagus detected on barium esophagograms: increased prevalence in patients with esophageal carcinoma. *Am J Roentgenol.* 1995; *165*(6): 1381–1385.
3. Teraishi F, Fujiwara T, Jikuhara A, et al. Esophageal intramural pseudodiverticulosis with esophageal strictures successfully treated with dilation therapy. *Ann Thorac Surg.* 2006; *82*(3): 1119–1121.

History

► 45-year-old man with solid and liquid dysphagia. He describes feeling food stick in the mid chest.

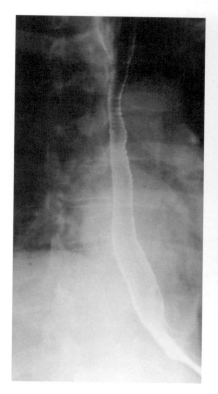 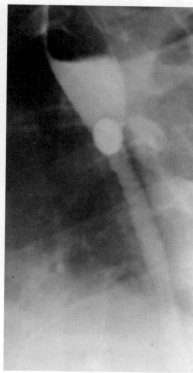

Case 7 Eosinophilic Esophagitis

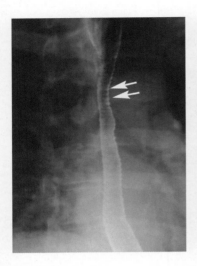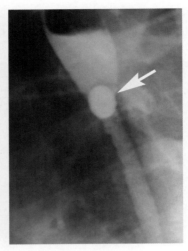

Findings

Double contrast esophagram shows smooth tapering of the proximal esophagus that leads to a narrowing of the mid esophagus (left image, arrows). The narrowed portion of the esophagus has concentric rings (left image, arrows), which resemble closely spaced tracheal rings. A 13 mm barium tablet (right image, arrow) lodges at the proximal edge of the narrowed segment.

Differential Diagnosis

▶ Peptic strictures: the transverse folds of peptic strictures are generally wider and do not extend more than halfway across the esophagus.
▶ Feline esophagus: the transverse striations in a feline esophagus are transient and not associated with a stricture.
▶ Nonperistaltic contractions of dysmotility: an irregular corrugated pattern that is transient and is not associated with a stricture.

Teaching Points

The prevalence of eosinophilic esophagitis is greater than previously thought. It is one of the most common causes of food impaction in the young adult population, typically affecting young men between 20 and 40 years of age with an allergic history or a family history of allergies. Most patients complain of long-standing dysphagia and frequent food impactions. The findings on barium evaluation of the esophagus are often diagnostic, but may be subtle. Esophageal strictures are the most common finding, often with distinctive ring-like indentations that produced a "ringed" esophagus. The rings or strictures may be of varying length and can be found throughout the esophagus. The rings may be difficult to visualize in the distended esophagus, and are better visualized on partially collapsed views. Eosinophilic esophagitis may also cause diffuse esophageal narrowing.

Management

The goal of treatment for eosinophilic esophagitis is to relieve symptoms of dysphagia. Gentle mechanical esophageal dilatation may be performed, and proton pump inhibitors and steroids may be used.

Further Readings

1. Zimmerman SL, Levine MS, Rubesin SE, et al. Idiopathic eosinophilic esophagitis in adults: the ringed esophagus. *Radiology.* 2005; 236: 159–165.
2. Vasilopoulos S, Murphy P, Auerbach A, et al. The small-caliber esophagus: an unappreciated cause of dysphagia for solids in patients with eosinophilic esophagitis. *Gastrointest Endosc.* 2002; 55: 99–106.

History

▶ 34-year-old woman with dysphagia.

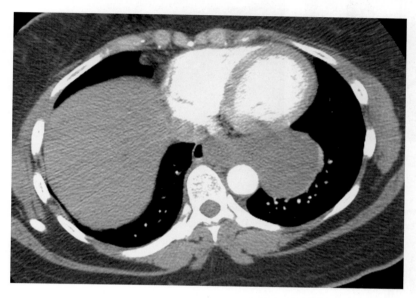

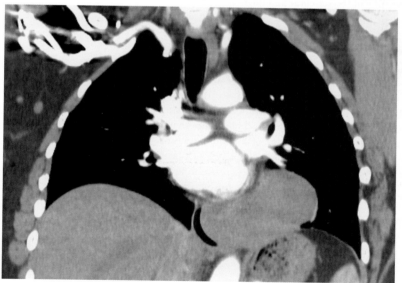

Case 8   Esophageal Duplication Cyst

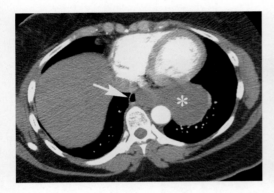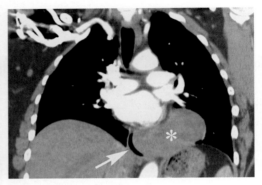

Findings

Contrast-enhanced CT shows a smoothly marginated homogeneous fluid-attenuation cyst (asterisk) that is inseparable from the distal esophageal wall. The cyst deviates the esophagus (arrows) to the right.

Differential Diagnosis

► Pericardial cyst: generally to the right of the heart without esophageal contact.
► Bronchogenic cyst: may show mural calcification.
► Meningocele: may show deformity of the vertebrae and intervertebral foramina.

Teaching Points

Cystic lesions of the lower thorax and upper abdomen are often congenital and include bronchogenic, duplication, neurenteric, and pericardial cysts. Esophageal foregut duplication cysts are uncommon and do not communicate with the esophageal lumen. These cysts may occur above or just below the diaphragm. Although they are often asymptomatic, duplication cysts may cause dysphagia or pain, and may hemorrhage or become infected. Most of these cysts are identified in infants and children, usually adjacent to the esophagus. Imaging findings of benign mediastinal cysts include a smooth margin with homogeneous fluid attenuation without internal enhancement or infiltration of adjacent structures. MRI may be more sensitive for identifying internal architecture. If clinically warranted, radionuclide imaging with Tc-99m pertechnetate may be useful to demonstrate ectopic gastric mucosa, which is present in up to 50 percent of duplication cysts in pediatric patients. If mural irregularity, irregular septations, or soft tissue components are seen, a teratoma or malignancy should be considered. Also, careful inspection of the vertebrae and intervertebral foramina should be made to exclude involvement of the central canal, such as may occur with a meningocele.

Management

Referral to surgery is appropriate since resection is curative. Unresected cysts enlarge over time, eventually producing symptoms related to mass effect on adjacent structures.

Further Reading

1. Jeung MY, Gasser B, Gangi A, Bogorin A, Charneau D, Wihlm JM, Dietemann JL, Roy C. Imaging of cystic masses of the mediastinum. *RadioGraphics*. 2002 Oct (22, special issue); S79–93.

History

▶ 34-year-old man with vague difficulty swallowing.

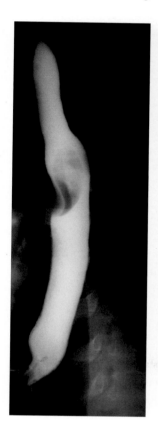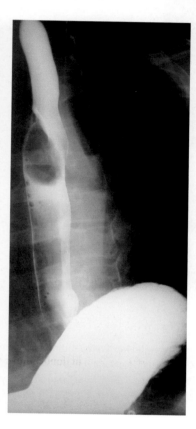

Case 9 Esophageal Leiomyoma

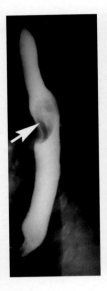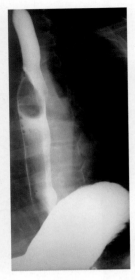

Findings

Esophagram shows a discrete mid-esophageal smooth oval filling defect (arrow) sharply outlined by barium. The lesion forms obtuse to right angles with the normal esophageal wall on the left image. This is characteristic of a submucosal lesion.

Differential Diagnosis

▶ Duplication cyst: may be indistinguishable from solid intramural tumors on barium swallow. Duplication cysts generally have a homogenous fluid attenuation on CT scans and high signal intensity on T2-weighted MR images.
▶ Lipoma: much less common submucosal esophageal lesion compared to leiomyomas. Esophagram may show a submucosal mass or a pedunculated, intraluminal mass. CT will show fat attenuation within a lipoma.
▶ Other less common submucosal lesions such as gastrointestinal stromal tumors, neurofibromas, hemangiomas, and fibromas may have a similar appearance to leiomyomas.

Teaching Points

Esophageal leiomyomas are the most common benign tumor of the esophagus. They occur twice as commonly in men as in women. The mean age at clinical presentation is 30 to 35 years. Many patients are asymptomatic, with lesions found incidentally. Dysphagia is the most common clinical complaint. Barium studies generally show a discrete, smoothly marginated submucosal mass that produces an obtuse or right angle with the wall of the esophagus when viewed in profile and an ovoid round or oval filling defect when viewed en face. Less commonly, leiomyomas may be multifocal or annular.

Management

Surgical excision (enucleation) of the tumor is recommended for those patients with symptomatic leiomyomas. Additionally, some authors recommend surgical resection of lesions greater than 5 cm. Asymptomatic patients and/or those with small lesions can be followed radiographically and/or endoscopically without adverse consequences; these lesions rarely cause bleeding and have little, if any, tendency to undergo sarcomatous degeneration.

Further Reading

1. Mutrie CJ, Donahue DM, Wain JC, et al. Esophageal leiomyoma: a 40-year experience. *Ann Thorac Surg.* 2005; *79*: 1122–1125.

History

▶ 52-year-old man with long history of gastroesophageal reflux complains of epigastric pain, several weeks of solid food dysphagia, and 20-pound weight loss over the past six months, secondary to anorexia.

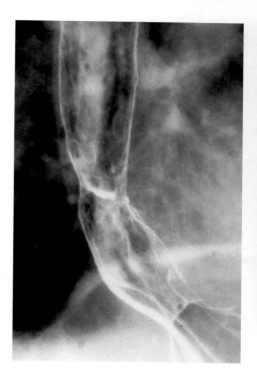
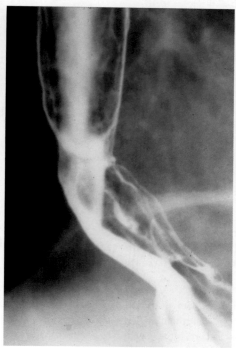

Case 10 Barrett Adenocarcinoma

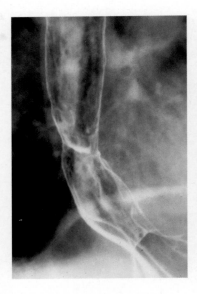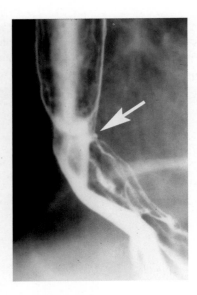

Findings

Double contrast esophagram shows a reticular mucosal pattern in the distal esophagus and a short irregular stricture with ulcerations (arrow) near the gastroesophageal junction. There is a small hiatal hernia.

Differential Diagnosis

► Peptic strictures: benign strictures are less likely to display abrupt change in caliber, focal irregularity, nodularity, or wall stiffening that is more commonly associated with malignant lesions.
► Squamous cell carcinoma: may not be distinguishable from adenocarcinoma radiographically, but tend to occur in the upper and middle portions of the esophagus. When they occur distally, they usually do not invade the stomach, which is more typical of adenocarcinoma.

Teaching Points

The incidence of esophageal adenocarcinoma is rising rapidly, particularly among men. A major risk factor for this disease is Barrett esophagus, a metaplastic change in the esophageal lining from squamous cell mucosa to an intestinal-type columnar mucosa as a result of long standing gastroesophageal reflux. Adenocarcinomas in Barrett esophagus may be infiltrating lesions that produce irregular esophageal strictures with nodularity and ulceration; intraluminal polypoid masses; ulcerative lesions; or varicoid lesions with submucosal tumor spread. Unlike squamous cancers, adenocarcinoma in Barrett has a tendency to invade the proximal stomach.

Management

Most patients with Barrett adenocarcinoma present with unresectable disease. In those patients presenting with early disease in which the cancer is limited to the mucosa, endoscopic resection is one potential therapy. Once the disease extends into the submucosa, however, the risk of lymph node metastases increases significantly and surgical resection combined with neoadjuvant or adjuvant radiation and/or chemotherapy is the treatment of choice.

Further Readings

1. Levine MS. Barrett esophagus: update for radiologists. *Abdom Imaging*. 2005 Mar-Apr; *30*(2): 133–141.
2. Sharma P. Clinical practice. Barrett's esophagus. *N Engl J Med*. 2009 Dec 24; *361*(26): 2548–2556.
3. Levine MS, Caroline D, Thompson JJ, et al. Adenocarcinoma of the esophagus: relationship to Barrett mucosa. *Radiology*. 1984 Feb; *150*(2): 305–309.

History

▶ 62-year-old man with severe chest pain and hypotension after vomiting.

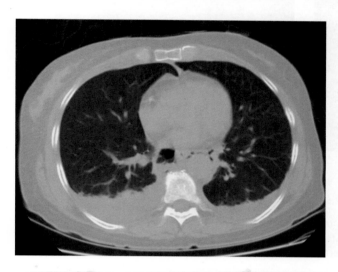

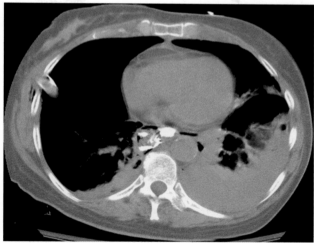

Case 11 Boerhaave Syndrome

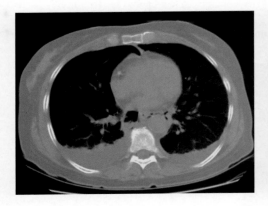 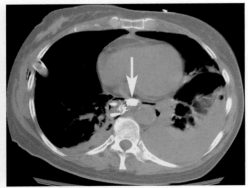

Findings

CT shows bilateral pleural effusions and pneumomediastinum anterior to the aorta and to the right of the esophagus. Subsequent CT with oral contrast shows dense contrast in the esophagus (arrow) and leakage into the irregular complex right mediastinal collection.

Differential Diagnosis

► Spontaneous pneumothorax: may occur in young healthy persons or those with underlying lung disease such as COPD, cystic fibrosis, prior pneumocystis pneumonia, or interstitial lung diseases. Mediastinal air is not seen.
► Spontaneous pneumomediastinum: rare and may present with chest pain and associated with asthma or COPD, or in intubated patients on positive pressure ventilation. Occasionally, may occur in otherwise healthy people.
► Spontaneous rupture of abnormal esophagus: esophageal perforation may occur with underlying esophageal malignancy or severe esophagitis.
► Iatrogenic perforation following endoscopy, dilatation, or surgery.

Teaching Points

Boerhaave syndrome, spontaneous rupture of the esophagus during vomiting, may occur following alcohol ingestion and large meal consumption. Rupture is typically located at the left supradiaphragmatic portion of the esophagus. Mackler triad of vomiting, severe chest pain, and subcutaneous emphysema is the classic clinical presentation. Unfortunately, most cases do not present with classic symptoms; therefore spontaneous esophageal rupture should be considered in any seriously ill patient with a combination of gastrointestinal and respiratory complaints. When Boerhaave syndrome is suspected, confirmation may be obtained with an esophagram with water soluble contrast or endoscopy, but false negative studies do occur. The most reliable CT finding is pneumomediastinum surrounding the distal esophagus. Additional findings may include esophageal wall thickening, pleural effusions, and pulmonary consolidations. If oral contrast is used, the CT may show the site of perforation and extraluminal extravasation of contrast.

Management

Boerhaave syndrome is a life-threatening condition requiring prompt treatment. Immediate surgery to repair the esophageal tear is the treatment of choice, but the use of esophageal stents and mediastinal drainage has been reported.

Further Reading

1. Ghanem N, Altehoefer C, Springer O, et. al. Radiological findings in Boerhaave's syndrome. *Emergency Radiol.* 2003; *10:* 8–13.

History

▶ 53-year-old man with chronic progressive chest pain after eating.

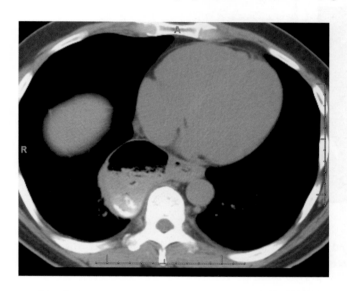

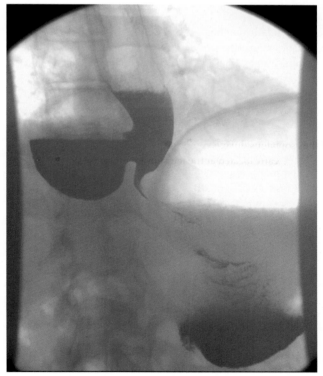

Case 12 Epiphrenic Diverticulum

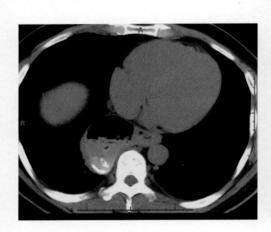 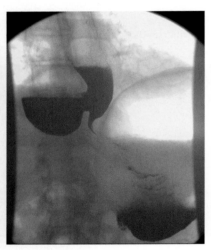

Findings

CT image shows oral contrast (left image) and air in a thin-walled outpouching to the right of the distal esophagus without surrounding fat. Esophagram (right image) shows communication of a large cavity with the lower esophagus.

Differential Diagnosis

► Hiatal hernia: almost always has thick gastric rugae and surrounding omental fat.
► Contained esophageal rupture: may be post-traumatic; occurs after violent retching or a complication of surgery or endoscopy and is generally suggested by the clinical history. No peristalsis of the extraluminal gas collection.

Teaching Points

Epiphrenic esophageal diverticula usually occur in middle-aged and elderly individuals who present with dysphagia, regurgitation, chest pain, or aspiration. Most esophageal diverticula are epiphrenic—that is, located near the diaphragm—and have a neck that is within 10 cm of the gastroesophageal junction, usually to the right side. Epiphrenic esophageal diverticula are associated with esophageal dysmotility disorders in 75 to 100 percent of patients; pulsion forces are commonly implicated in the pathogenesis. Weight loss, gastrointestinal bleeding, or even cancer may result from esophageal diverticula. Esophagram is the best exam to define the location and size of the neck of the diverticulum, the overall dimensions of the outpouching, and the severity of esophageal dysmotility and retention of material in the diverticulum. Dysmotility and retention of material are less easily tested at cross section imaging or endoscopy.

Management

Minimally invasive techniques are becoming commonplace for symptomatic diverticula. Excision of the diverticulum is often performed with an associated longitudinal myotomy to decrease intraluminal esophageal pressures. Post-surgical morbidity relates to persistent esophageal dysmotility, suture leakage, or diverticulum recurrence.

Further Readings

1. Soares R, Herbella FA, Prachand VN, Ferguson MK, & Patti MG. Epiphrenic diverticulum of the esophagus. From pathophysiology to treatment. *J Gastrointest Surg.* 2010 Dec; *14*(12): 2009–2015.
2. Fasano NC, Levine MS, Rubesin SE, Redfern RO, & Laufer I. Epiphrenic diverticulum: clinical and radiographic findings in 27 patients. *Dysphagia.* 2003; 18: 9–15.

History

▶ 70-year-old man with epigastric pain.

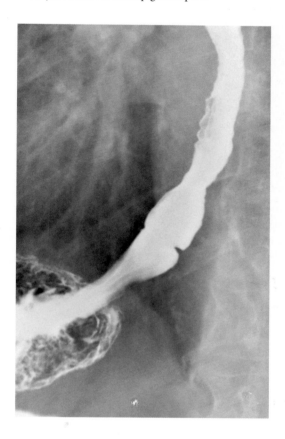

Case 13 Hiatal Hernia

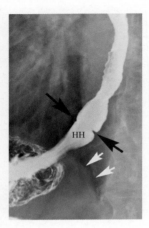

Findings

Rugal folds of the proximal stomach extend above the diaphragm (white arrows) forming a small hiatal hernia (labeled HH). The gastroesophageal junction is above the diaphragm, demarcated as a ring-like defect called the B-ring (black arrows), marks the proximal extent of the hiatal hernia and the gastroesophageal junction. Tertiary contractions of the esophagus are present.

Differential Diagnosis

▶ Peptic stricture: ring-like peptic strictures may occur. They have broader vertical height than a B-ring or Schatzki ring and tapered margins.

▶ Distal esophageal webs: occur in the setting of reflux scarring and are usually associated with a peptic stricture.

▶ Schatzki ring: symptomatic B-ring.

▶ A-ring: a transiently contractile ring in the distal esophagus located proximal to the B-ring. It demarcates the proximal margin of the esophageal vestibule.

Teaching Points

Sliding hiatal hernias are defined as extensions of the gastroesophageal junction, and therefore a portion of the stomach, above the diaphragm. Observation of the lower esophageal ring above the diaphragmatic hiatus—or gastric folds above the diaphragm when the lower esophageal ring is not seen—establishes the diagnosis. Paraesophageal hernias are much less common and are defined by herniation of a portion of the stomach through the esophageal hiatus, alongside the distal esophagus but with the gastroesophageal junction in its normal position. Mixed hernias also may occur.

   Lower esophageal mucosal rings, also known as B-rings, are the most common ring-like narrowing of the distal esophagus. The B-ring corresponds to the location of the squamocolumnar junction. The ring is a smooth and symmetric linear, ring-like defect in the distal esophagus. It is a fixed, reproducible finding with well-defined margins and a height of 2 to 4 mm.

Management

Sliding hiatal hernias may be associated with gastroesophageal reflux. Large, symptomatic sliding hernias may require surgical correction. In contrast, all paraesophageal hernias should be corrected because they are prone to volvulus and obstruction as they enlarge.

Further Reading

1. Smith DF, Ott DJ, Gelfand DW, & Chen MY. Lower esophageal mucosal ring: correlation of referred symptoms with radiographic findings using a marshmallow bolus. *Am J Roentgenol.* 1998; *171*(5): 1361–1365.

History

▶ 35-year-old man with progressive dysphagia.

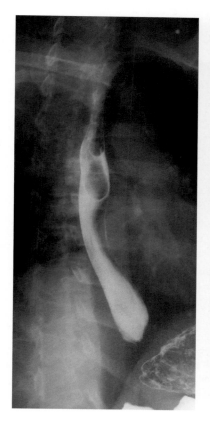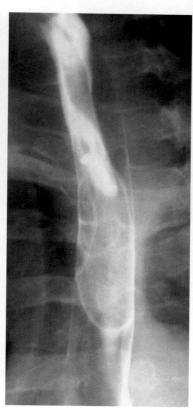

Case 14 Giant Fibrovascular Polyp

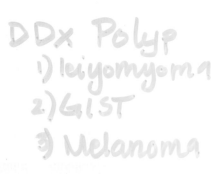

*DDx Polyp
1) leiyomyoma
2) GIST
3) Melanoma*

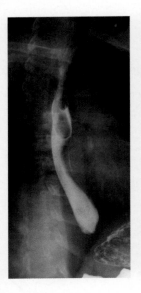
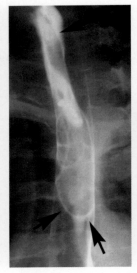
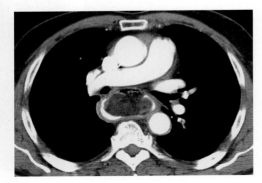

Findings

Barium esophagram shows an elongated, expansile, sausage-shaped intraluminal mass in the proximal esophagus. Barium flows around the contours of the intraluminal mass (arrows). The CT scan from a different patient with a fibrovascular polyp shows fat attenuation within the polyp and expansion of the esophagus around the polyp.

Differential Diagnosis

► Polypoid intraluminal tumors: benign and malignant tumors of the esophagus such as leiomyoma, gastrointestinal stromal tumors, and melanoma metastasis may have an intraluminal polypoid component.

► Foreign body: impacted foreign bodies such as hot dogs or other meat impactions may have an elongated appearance. A clinical history suggesting food impaction is usually present.

Teaching Points

Fibrovascular polyps are unusual, benign esophageal tumors that arise in the cervical esophagus at the level of the cricopharyngeus. These tumors grow slowly and elongate over time, extending into the middle and distal esophagus by the time the patient complains of symptoms. The majority of patients complain of slowly progressive dysphagia. Other symptoms include weight loss, bleeding from ulcerations on the polyp, and asphyxia from regurgitation of the polyp into the mouth or laryngeal compression. Esophagram classically shows an intraluminal, sausage-shaped mass extending from the cervical esophagus. The site of origin in the cervical esophagus is usually not visualized on esophagram. On CT, the mass is typically heterogeneous in attenuation and contains fat.

Management

Cervical esophagotomy with exploration and resection of the mass and the pedicle is the procedure of choice. If the lesion is very large and extends to the distal esophagus, a thoracotomy may be necessary.

Further Readings

1. Levine MS, Buck J, Pantongrag-Brown L, et al. Fibrovascular polyps of the esophagus: clinical, radiographic, and pathologic findings in 16 patients. *Am J Roentgenol.* 1996; *166*: 781–787.
2. Solerio D, Gasparri G, Ruffini E., et al. Giant fibrovascular polyp of the esophagus. *Dis Esophagus.* 2005; *18*: 410–412.

History

► 55-year-old man with dysphagia.

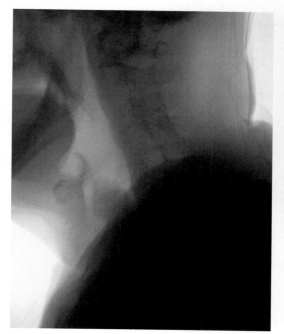
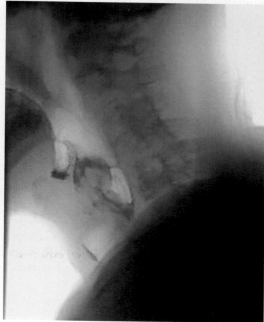

Case 15 Pharyngeal Carcinoma

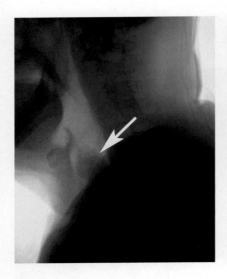 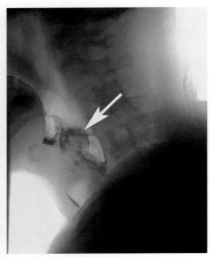

Findings

Scout (left) lateral fluoroscopic image of the neck shows a soft tissue bulge (arrow) along the anterior hypopharynx below the level of the epiglottis. Image obtained after oral barium administration (right image) confirms a rounded mass coated by barium (arrow).

Differential Diagnosis

► Impacted food: generally, patient has history of recent eating with sudden trapped food. Further evaluation is needed after mechanical food removal to exclude an underlying esophageal process.
► Fibroepithelial polyp: usually arises posteriorly just distal to the cricopharyngeus. Symptoms are chronic.

Teaching Points

Cancers of the pharynx and hypopharynx are usually squamous cell carcinoma; risk factors include smoking, alcohol consumption, and Asian ethnicity. It is unusual to find a malignancy as a cause of dysphagia in a swallowing study, but because of the profound effect of this diagnosis on patients, malignancy should be considered. Pharyngeal carcinomas may occur in a younger population than other causes of aspiration, such as dementia, stroke, or demyelinating diseases. Most patients with pharyngeal and hypopharyngeal squamous cell carcinomas have recent onset of symptoms, including hoarseness and dysphagia. The overall five-year survival rate for these patients is 20 to 40 percent.

At imaging, careful inspection of the contours of the epiglottis, valleculae, and aryepiglottic folds helps to identify unusual thickening or contour bulges caused by cancer. The affected mucosa may show granular, nodular, ulcerated, or lobulated contours. The finding of fixation/non-movement/non-distension of a wall of the hypopharynx may suggest the presence of an infiltrative tumor.

Management

If a tumor is suspected, direct visualization and biopsy allow a definitive diagnosis. Local staging by CT or MRI prior to resection or radiotherapy is useful because local invasion or lymphadenopathy may be present in 70 percent of patients.

Further Reading

1. Mong A, Levine MS, Rubenstein SE, and Laufer I. Epigottic carcinoma as a cause of laryngeal penetration and aspiration. *Am J Roentgenol.* 2003 Jan; *180*(1): 207–211.

History

▶ 55-year-old man complains of halitosis.

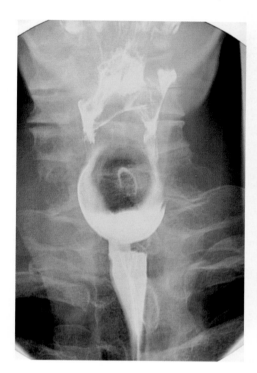 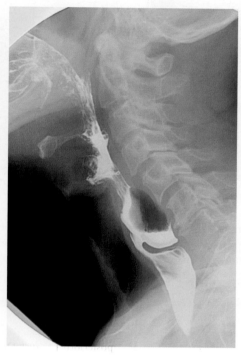

Case 16 Zenker Diverticulum

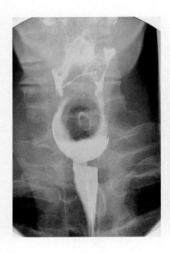
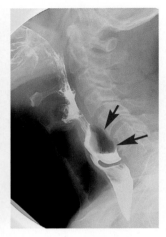
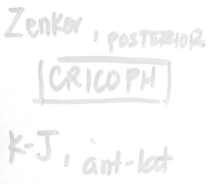

Findings

Esophagram shows an air and barium-filled saccular pouch on the anterior-posterior view that projects posteriorly on the lateral view (arrows) and deviates the lumen of the pharynx anteriorly. The pouch bulges posteriorly and is located immediately above the cricopharyngeus muscle.

Differential Diagnosis

► Killian-Jamieson diverticulum: occurs below the level of the cricopharyngeus muscle and projects anteriorly and laterally to the proximal cervical esophagus.
► Pseudo-Zenker diverticulum: occurs when barium is trapped above the cricopharyngeus muscle. Unlike a true Zenker diverticulum, it does not protrude posteriorly to the pharynx.

Teaching Points

Zenker diverticulum, also known as posterior hypopharyngeal diverticulum or pouch, is the most common pharyngeal diverticulum. It occurs at an area of anatomic weakness called Killian triangle, which is located in the posterior wall of the distal pharynx where there is divergence of cricopharyngeal muscle fibers from the inferior pharyngeal constrictor. The exact etiology of Zenker diverticulum is unknown; however it is considered to be a pulsion diverticulum that arises from a failure of the cricopharyngeus muscle to relax during swallowing. Patients are usually in their seventh and eighth decades of life and may be asymptomatic or may complain of halitosis, dysphagia, regurgitation of undigested food, hoarseness, chronic cough, or recurrent pneumonia. Occasionally, Zenker diverticulum will be apparent on radiography as a soft tissue mass in the retrotracheal region and may contain an air fluid level. In barium studies, Zenker diverticulum projects posteriorly from the distal pharynx just above the level of the cricopharyngeus muscle. A large diverticulum may extend downward and laterally and compress the proximal cervical esophagus.

Management

Traditionally, surgery has been performed on patients with symptomatic Zenker diverticulum. More recently, endoscopic treatments with flexible endoscopes offer less invasive therapeutic options.

Further Readings

1. Rubesin SE. Pharynx. In: Laufer I, Levine MS. *Double contrast gastrointestinal radiology*. 2nd ed. Philadelphia: Saunders, 1992: 73–105.
2. Rubesin SE, Levine MS. Killian-Jamieson diverticula: radiographic findings in 16 patients. *Am J Roentgenol*. 2001; *177*(1): 85–89.

Part 2   Stomach

History

► 74-year-old man with several weeks of epigastric pain and guaiac-positive stools. Upper endoscopy was negative to the level of the duodenal bulb.

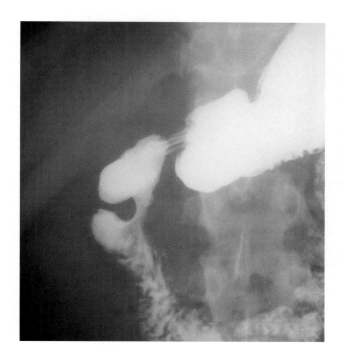

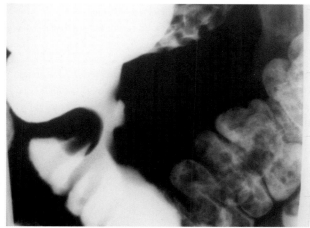

Case 17   Peptic Ulcer

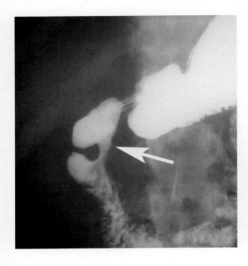
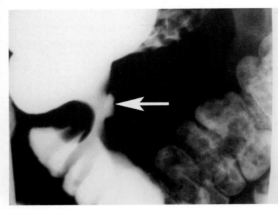

Findings

Prone image (left image) from an upper gastrointestinal series shows a prominent eccentric lateral narrowing (incisura) of the post-bulbar duodenum. A faint collection of gas and contrast (arrow) opposite the narrowing suggests a posterior wall ulcer. Subsequent oblique supine view (right image) of the post-bulbar duodenum shows barium filling the posterior ulcer (arrow) with under-cutting of the mucosa by the ulcer crater.

Differential Diagnosis

▶ Annular pancreas: smooth extrinsic narrowing of the second portion of the duodenum. Most commonly found prenatally, during infancy, or in childhood; adults with annular pancreas may be asymptomatic or develop pancreatitis or duodenal obstruction.
▶ Pancreatic cancer: may narrow the duodenum with sparing of the ampulla (inverted "3" sign).
▶ Other: post-bulbar strictures may uncommonly result from peptic ulcer disease or, rarely. Crohn disease.

Teaching Points

Peptic ulcers occurring in the post-bulbar duodenum account for approximately 5 to 10 percent of duodenal ulcers, but the incidence of associated upper gastrointestinal bleeding and massive hemorrhage is much higher in peptic than in bulbar ulcers. Post-bulbar ulcers are much more common in men and older people than bulbar ulcers, and the symptoms are often nonspecific; typically the pain radiates to various locations including the upper abdomen, flanks, and back. Post-bulbar ulcers may be more difficult to diagnose clinically, endoscopically, and radiographically than bulbar ulcers. The most striking radiological finding is a prominent infolding of the duodenal wall—the incisura—caused by spasm and edema. The area opposite the incisura should be carefully evaluated for the ulcer.

Management

Post-bulbar ulcers are managed as other peptic ulcers with therapy for *helicobacter pylori* and proton pump inhibitors. Intervention may be necessary for massive bleeding or strictures.

Further Readings

1. Carucci LR, Levine MS, Rubesin SE, Laufer I. Upper gastrointesintal tract barium examination of postbulbar duodenal ulcers. *Am J Roentgenol*. 2004; *182*: 927–930.
2. Jayaraman MV, Mayo-Smith WW, Movson JS, et. al. CT of the duodenum: an overlooked segment gets its due. *RadioGraphics*. 2001; *21*: S147–S160.

History

▶ 66-year-old woman presents with worsening upper abdominal pain.

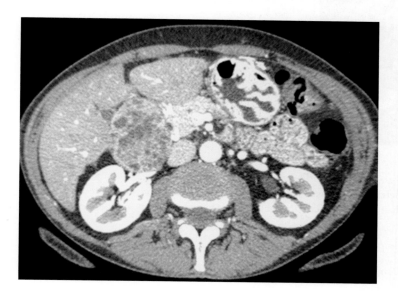

Case 18 Zollinger-Ellison Syndrome

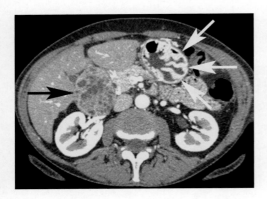

Findings

Contrast-enhanced CT shows a heterogeneous mass (black arrow) involving the duodenum and pancreatic head without pancreatic or bile duct dilatation. Gastric rugal folds are hyperenhancing and thickened (white arrows).

Differential Diagnosis

► Gastrointestinal stromal tumor: may form a large non-obstructive mass in the duodenum, but is not usually associated with gastric fold thickening.
► Lymphoma: masses are usually homogeneous at CT and are usually associated with prominent lymphadenopathy.
► Extra-adrenal paragangliomas are commonly hypervascular and non-obstructive, and clinical symptoms or the presence of urine metanephrines can be suggestive of the diagnosis.

Teaching Points

Zollinger-Ellison syndrome is a complex condition involving hypersecretion of gastrin, which can lead to peptic ulcers. Patients with this syndrome show an elevated fasting serum gastrin in the presence of hyperchlorhydria or an acidic gastric pH ≤ 2. Most patients with Zollinger-Ellison syndrome have gastrinomas, functional pancreatic endocrine tumors that are most frequently found in the gastrinoma triangle demarcated by the pancreatic neck, junction of the cystic and common bile duct, and third portion of the duodenum. Gastrinomas and insulinomas are the most common pancreatic endocrine tumors. At the time of discovery both tumors tend to be smaller than other endocrine tumors due to symptoms related to hormone hypersecretion. Both tumors may be hypervascular. For these reasons, evaluation at CT and MRI is best obtained with multiphase imaging and thin sections. Somatostatin receptor scintigraphy may also help localize lesions and metastases. Large endocrine tumors of the pancreas and duodenum do not generally obstruct the pancreatic or bile duct. Gastrinomas may also occur in multiple endocrine neoplasia syndrome type 1 or may be sporadic.

Management

Medications such as proton pump inhibitors may alleviate the symptoms of gastrin hypersecretion. Surgical resection may be curative. Preoperative identification of liver metastases is critical to guide the decision to pursue pancreatic and bowel resection of the primary tumor.

Further Reading

1. Horton KM, Hruban RH, Yeo C, Fishman EK. Multi-detector row CT of pancreatic islet cell tumors. *RadioGraphics*. 2006; *26*(2): 453–464.

History

▶ 55-year-old man with epigastric pain, weight loss, nausea, and leg edema.

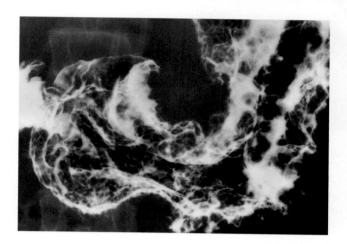

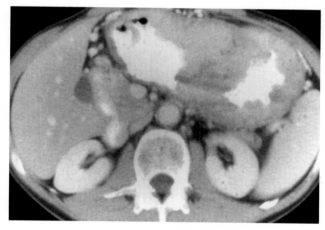

Case 19 Ménétrier Disease

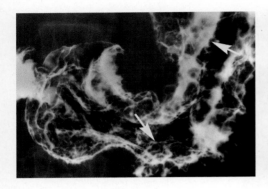 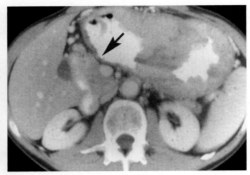

Findings

Spot image of the stomach (left image) shows thick gastric folds, most notably in the fundus and body. Thin linear collections of contrast (white arrows) are present between the thickened folds. CT (right image) shows large lobulated folds and wall thickening in the gastric body. The antrum has normal wall thickness (black arrow).

Differential Diagnosis

► Zollinger-Ellison syndrome: gastric and duodenal ulcers are often present in addition to gastric, duodenal, and jejunal fold thickening. A gastrin-secreting tumor (gastrinoma) may be located in the pancreas or duodenum.

► *H. pylori* gastritis: common cause of antral fold thickening, but the degree of thickening is considerably less.

► Lymphoma: may be indistinguishable from other causes of fold thickening on barium exams. CT may show extragastric findings such as enlarged lymph nodes and splenomegaly.

► Varices: tortuous submucosal filling defects. Fundic varices are typically posteriomedial and may be associated with esophageal varices.

Teaching Points

Ménétrier disease is a rare disease that has a bimodal age distribution. The childhood form, more common in boys, is linked to CMV infection and often resolves spontaneously, unlike the adult form. The adult form, also more common in males, is thought to involve improper regulation of the epidermal growth factor receptor signaling pathway. Marked gastric mucosal hypertrophy secondary to hyperplasia of superficial mucosal epithelial cells leads to the characteristic large lobulated gastric folds. Giant rugal folds are most prominent along the greater curvature and tend to spare the antrum and cardia. Albumin loss across the gastric mucosa occurs at a high rate and is not only responsible for the clinical manifestation of peripheral edema, but also for intravascular hypovolemia which may account for the increased incidence of thrombotic events in Ménétrier disease. The associated risk for gastric malignancy remains unclear.

Management

Proton pump inhibitors and steroids show varying benefit. Gastrectomy offers a proven benefit in patients with severe symptoms.

Further Reading

1. Friedman J, Platnick J, Farruggia S, Khilko N, Mody K, Tyshkov M. Best cases from the AFIP: ménétrier disease. *RadioGraphics*. 2009; *29*: 297–301.

History

▶ 24-year-old man with abdominal pain and hematemesis.

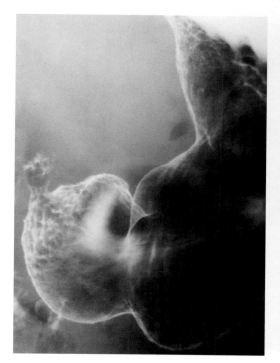
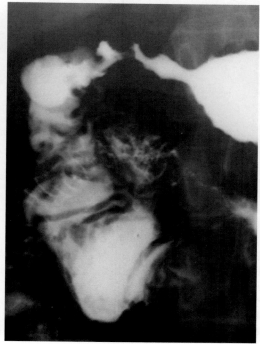

Case 20 Crohn Disease

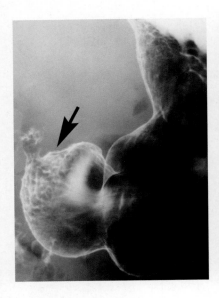 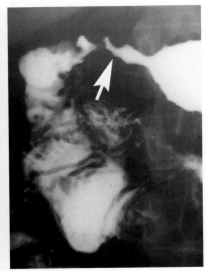

Findings

Upper gastrointestinal series shows nodularity of the gastric antral mucosa (left image, arrow) with a cobblestone pattern and multiple small ulcers. The pylorus and duodenal bulb are narrowed, deformed, and ulcerated (right image, arrow).

Differential Diagnosis

► Gastric tuberculosis: may be indistinguishable from Crohn disease. Usually secondary to pulmonary tuberculosis, therefore correlation with chest radiographs and clinical history is helpful.
► Gastric sarcoidosis: rare location for sarcoidosis and should be considered only when systemic disease is present.

Teaching Points

Crohn disease is an idiopathic chronic inflammatory bowel disease that may affect any part of the gastrointestinal tract. The hallmarks of Crohn disease include segmental and transmural inflammation. Crohn disease primarily affects the ileum and colon; gastroduodenal involvement occurs in only 1 to 13 percent of these patients. Isolated gastroduodenal Crohn disease is quite rare. Although many Crohn patients may have granulomas on biopsy from the stomach and duodenum, only a small percentage will have symptomatic disease. Symptoms attributable to gastroduodenal disease include epigastric pain and nausea/vomiting secondary to ulceration and stricture. Upper endoscopy usually reveals mucosal edema with multiple raised erosions throughout the gastric antrum and duodenum as well as luminal narrowing.

Management

The majority of patients diagnosed with symptomatic gastroduodenal Crohn disease will be managed medically. Medications aimed at suppressing acid production and inflammation are the cornerstone of treatment. Obstruction is the primary indication for surgery, but only 10 to 20 percent of patients presenting with obstructive symptoms will require surgical intervention.

Further Readings

1. Tremaine WJ. Gastroduodenal Crohn's disease: medical management. *Inflamm Bowel Dis.* 2003 Mar; 9(2): 127–128.
2. van Hogezand RA, Witte AM, Veenendaal RA, Wagtmans MJ, and Lamers CB. Proximal Crohn's disease: review of the clinicopathologic features and therapy. *Inflamm Bowel Dis.* 2001; 7(4): 328–337.

History

▶ 75-year-old man with a history of recent abdominal surgery presents to the emergency room complaining of severe abdominal pain. Patient is found to be hypotensive and tachycardic.

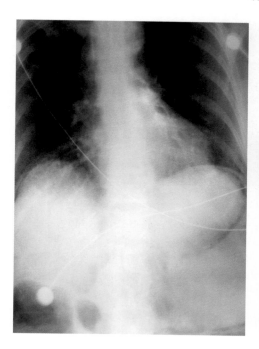

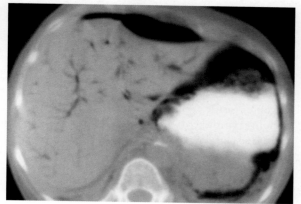

Case 21 Emphysematous Gastritis

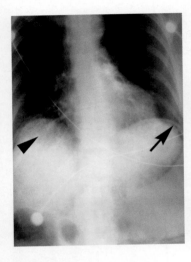
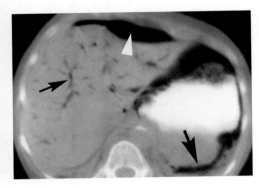

Findings

Abdominal radiograph (left image) shows an curvilinear lucency in the left upper quadrant (arrow), suggesting gastric pneumatosis and/or free intraperitoneal air. There is also gas in the in the portal veins of the liver (arrowhead). CT (right image) shows gas infiltrating throughout a thickened gastric wall (large arrow) and portal venous gas (small arrow). Additionally, a large amount of free intraperitoneal air is present (arrowhead).

Differential Diagnosis

▸ Benign gastric emphysema: intramural air is more linear in its distribution and the gastric mucosal wall is not thickened. May occur after severe coughing or vomiting or may be iatrogenic from nasogastric tube insertion or endoscopy.
▸ Gastric bezoar: air in the interstices or aggregated ingested fibrous material within the lumen of the stomach.

Teaching Points

Emphysematous gastritis is a rare entity that is defined by the presence of intramural air due to infection by microorganisms such as *Streptococci*, *E. coli*, *Enterobacter* species, and *S. aureus*. No age or gender preference exists, and the mortality rate approaches 80 percent. Normally the stomach is quite resistant to invasion from local and systemic infection secondary to its acidic pH, abundant blood supply, and the intrinsic characteristics of its mucosa. Predisposing factors for superinfection include ingestion of corrosive substances, alcoholism, recent abdominal surgery, trauma, and gastric volvulus. Characteristic imaging findings consist of an irregular and nodular pattern of pneumatosis and thickened mucosal folds. In the most severe cases, pneumoperitoneum and portal venous gas may be present. Emesis of a necrotic cast of the stomach is clinically pathognomic for this disease.

Management

Management of emphysematous gastritis requires intense supportive care and early administration of broad-spectrum antibiotics. Surgical intervention in the acute phase is often delayed until the patient is stabilized, unless perforation has occurred.

Further Reading

1. Grayson DE, Abbott RM, Levy AD, Sherman PM. Emphysematous Infections of the Abdomen and Pelvis: A Pictorial Review. *RadioGraphics*. 2002; *22*: 543–561.

History

▶ 27-year-old man with repeated episodes of vomiting and several months of early satiety.

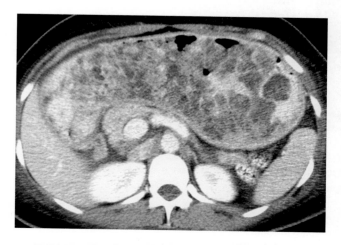

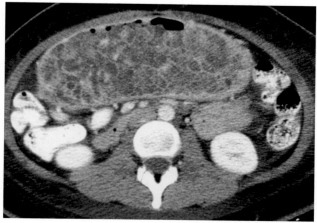

Case 22 Juvenile Polyposis Syndrome

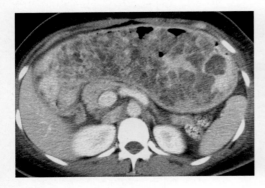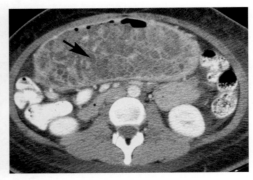

Findings

CT shows innumerable hypodense polypoid lesions in the stomach. Some have peripheral enhancement (right image, arrow). The gastric wall is normal thickness.

Differential Diagnosis

▶ Peutz-Jeghers syndrome and multiple hamartoma syndrome (Cowden disease): these syndromes are usually associated with mucocutaneous lesions.
▶ Cronkhite-Canada syndrome: polyps are frequently sessile and usually smaller in size.
▶ Familial adenomatous polyposis (Gardner syndrome): polyps are predominantly located within the gastric body and fundus, and all patients have colonic polyps.

Teaching Points

Juvenile polyposis syndrome is an extremely rare autosomal dominant disease that typically presents early in life and carries a high mortality rate. Several subtypes exist including juvenile polyposis coli and juvenile polyposis of infancy, both of which may present with intussusception, diarrhea, and recurrent gastrointestinal bleeding. A third subtype, termed diffuse juvenile polyposis, may cause gastric obstruction and protein-losing enteropathy. Juvenile polyposis syndrome may be diagnosed if the patient has more than five juvenile polyps in the colorectum, multiple juvenile polyps throughout the gastrointestinal tract, or any number of juvenile polyps and a family history of juvenile polyps. After the colon, the stomach is most often affected by the hamartomatous polyps of juvenile polyposis syndrome. Several hundred polyps may be present at diagnosis, with the gastric polyps predominantly occurring in the antrum. Juvenile polyposis syndrome carries an increased risk of gastrointestinal malignancy, with cancers occurring in the colon and stomach.

Management

If the patient has a small number of polyps, the disease burden typically is managed with polypectomy. Extremely large numbers of polyps may require gastrectomy, but clinical symptoms dictate treatment. Radiologists should be aware of the common extraintestinal manifestations of juvenile polyposis syndrome; these include cardiac anomalies and pulmonary arteriovenous malformations.

Further Reading

1. Covarrubias DJ, Huprich JE. Best cases from the AFIP. Juvenile polyposis of the stomach. *RadioGraphics*. 2002; *22*(2): 415–420.

History

▶ 65-year-old man with gastrointestinal bleeding, nausea and vomiting.

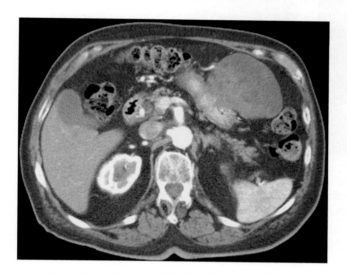

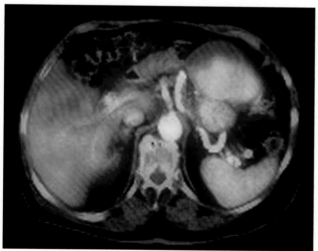

Case 23 Gastrointestinal Stromal Tumor (GIST)

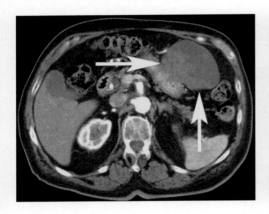 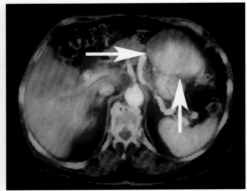

Findings

CT (left image) shows a large, well circumscribed, heterogeneously enhancing exophytic mass along the anterior stomach (arrows). Fused PET/CT (right image) shows marked FDG-avidity in the mass (arrows).

Differential Diagnosis

▶ Gastric lymphoma: often has prominent associated lymphadenopathy and tends to appear more homogeneous in attenuation.
▶ Gastric adenocarcinoma: more commonly infiltrative with wall-thickening and may limit gastric distensibility.
▶ Metastasis: patients usually have a known primary malignancy.
▶ Other mesenchymal tumors such as leiomyoma, carcinoid, leiomyoblastoma.

Teaching Points

Gastrointestinal stromal tumors (GISTs) are uncommon tumors that can occur anywhere in the gastrointestinal tract, but appear most commonly in the stomach. Patients may present with an enlarging abdominal mass, hematemesis or melena. GISTs can be seen at any age, but peak in the sixth and seventh decades of life and show no sex predilection. These tumors are typically solitary and submucosal with exophytic or, less commonly, endoluminal extension. Tumor necrosis, ulceration, and calcification are common. Metastases tend to involve the liver and peritoneal cavity. Both the primary lesion and metastases tend to be FDG-avid, and PET has been shown to be helpful in monitoring early therapy response. Like lymphomas, but unlike adenocarcinomas, GIST tumors tend not to obstruct bowel, blood vessels, or bile ducts until they grow large in size.

Management

Surgical resection is the best chance of cure for malignant GIST. Tyrosine kinase inhibitors such as imatinib are used to treat metastatic and recurrent GIST and can cause cystic change, decreased contrast enhancement, and diminished uptake of F-18-fluorodeoxyglucose in these tumors. Many tumors eventually develop resistance to imatinib.

Further Readings

1. Burkill GJC, Badran M, Al-Muderis O, Thomas JM, Judson IR, Fisher C, Moskovic EC. Malignant gastrointestinal stromal tumor: distribution, imaging features, and pattern of metastatic spread. *Radiology*. 2003 Feb; *226*: 527–532.
2. Gayed I, Vu T, Iyer R, Johnson M, Macapinlac H, Swanston N, Podoloff D. The role of 18F-FDG PET in staging and early prediction of response to therapy of recurrent gastrointestinal stromal tumors. *J Nucl Med*. 2004 Jan; *45*(1): 17–21.

History

► 55-year-old man with vague abdominal pain and mild dyspepsia.

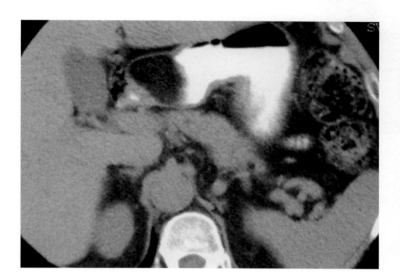

Case 24 Gastric Lipoma

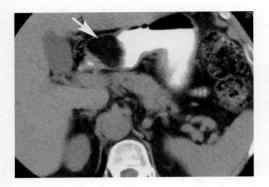

Findings

CT shows a rounded mass in the gastric antrum (arrow) with smooth margins. This mass is uniformly hypodense with an attenuation value consistent with fatty tissue.

Differential Diagnosis

▶ Liposarcoma: extremely rare, large exophytic masses. Areas of heterogeneous fatty density, liquefaction secondary to myxoid degeneration, necrosis, or hemorrhage may be present.

▶ Teratoma: uncommon childhood tumor that is usually exogastric. The mass is often complex, containing fat, fluid, and calcifications.

Teaching Points

Lipomas are rare gastric masses composed of well differentiated adipose tissue surrounded by a fibrous capsule. They occur more frequently in older patients. Lipomas usually present as solitary masses and are found most often in the gastric antrum. The majority of gastric lipomas are present in the submucosa and are rarely subserosal in origin. Subserosal lipomas are rarely symptomatic, but submucosal masses larger than 3 cm may present with pain, obstruction, and acute or chronic hemorrhage secondary to pressure necrosis with subsequent ulceration. Malignant transformation of gastric lipomas has not been reported.

Management

Definitive diagnosis with CT is possible and precludes the need for endoscopic biopsy. Surgical intervention is indicated when symptoms are life-threatening or unremitting or when malignancy cannot be excluded. If asymptomatic, a proven lipoma requires no further intervention.

Further Readings

1. Ferrozzi F, Tognini G, Bova D, Pavone P. Lipomatous tumors of the stomach: CT findings and differential diagnosis. *J Comput Assist Tomogr*. 2000; *24*: 854–858.
2. Thompson WM, Kende AI, Levy AD. Imaging characteristics of gastic lipomas in 16 adult and pediatric patients. *Am J Roentgenol* 2003; *181*: 981–985.

History

▶ 67-year-old woman with epigastric pain.

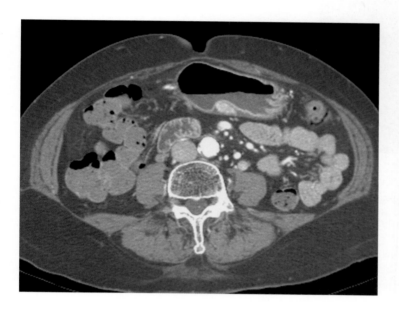

Case 25 Ectopic Pancreas

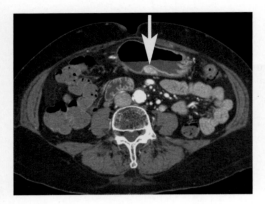

Findings

Contrast-enhanced CT image shows a small, heterogeneously enhancing, flat, oval submucosal mass (arrow) in the gastric antrum.

Differential Diagnosis

▶ Submucosal mesenchymal tumor: gastrointestinal stromal tumor (GIST), lipoma, leiomyoma, glomus tumor, schwannoma, and carcinoid tumors originate in the submucosa. Most may ulcerate. Gastric lipoma can be diagnosed by the presence of macroscopic fat.

▶ Submucosal metastatic tumor: patients with gastric metastasis have a known primary malignancy. Melanoma, breast, lung, lymphoma, and Kaposi sarcoma are the most common primaries to metastasize to the stomach.

▶ Submucosal gastric carcinoma: gastric carcinoma appearing isolated focally in the submucosa is rare. Central ulceration may occur.

Teaching Points

Pancreatic tissue may occur heterotopically (less than 2 percent of autopsy series), typically within a few centimeters of the gastroduodenal junction in the stomach, sometimes in the duodenum and occasionally in the more distal small bowel. Also known as a pancreatic rest, an ectopic pancreas is usually an incidental finding. Rare complications include pancreatitis, pseudocyst, pancreatic tumor, gastric outlet or intestinal obstruction, bile duct obstruction, and intussusception. Most pancreatic rests are less than 2 cm and grow very slowly if at all. Many cases will show central "dimpling" or umbilication on UGI or endoscopy and occasionally may show a rudimentary pancreatic duct. CT and endoluminal ultrasound both show fine irregularity of the margins. Ultrasound shows heterogeneous glandular morphology as opposed to a neoplastic process, which is often well defined and homogeneous. Prominent enhancement of overlying mucosa may be present, likely due to inflammatory changes in the underlying pancreatic rest. An ectopic pancreas usually follows the signal intensity (MRI) and attenuation (CT) of the normal pancreas on all sequences.

Management

Incidental small submucosal lesions that show characteristic findings of ectopic pancreas do not require further work-up. Since endoscopic biopsy of these lesions often shows nonspecific findings, surgical or endoscopic resection may be needed.

Further Reading

1. Kim JY, Lee JM, Kim KW, et al. Ectopic pancreas: CT findings with emphasis on differentiation from small gastrointestinal stromal tumor and leiomyoma. *Radiology*. 2009; *252*(1): 92–100.

History

▶ 60-year-old man with three months of progressive weight loss, early satiety, and worsening epigastric pain.

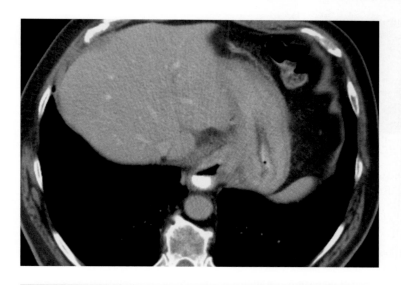

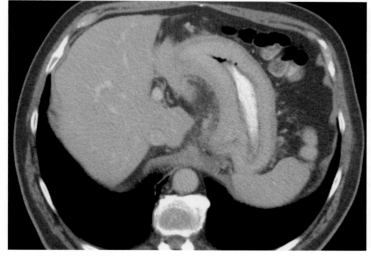

Case 26 Gastric Adenocarcinoma Producing Linitis Plastica

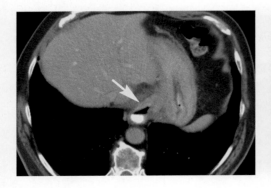 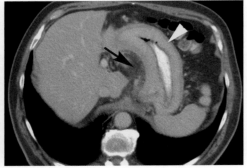

Findings

CT shows a diffusely thickened, homogeneously enhancing gastric wall (arrowhead). The wall thickening extends to involve the distal esophagus (white arrow). Linear stranding is present in the perigastric fat (black arrow).

Differential Diagnosis

► Gastric lymphoma: often causes homogeneous thickening of the gastric wall. Perigastric fat planes are usually preserved, and bulky lymph nodes may be present.

► Metastatic disease: breast cancer metastasis may produce a similar linitis plastica pattern that is identical to primary gastric adenocarcinoma.

► Ménétrier disease: the thick gastric folds of Ménétrier disease are usually most prominent within the gastric fundus and body. Linear collections of contrast between thickened rugal folds are often present.

Teaching Points

Adenocarcinoma represents approximately 95 percent of all gastric malignancies and usually occurs in the fifth or sixth decade of life. Prognosis depends upon the tumor stage at the time of diagnosis. Five-year survival rates decrease from 90 percent in early stage disease to less than 20 percent in advanced malignancy. CT is the imaging modality of choice for locoregional gastric cancer staging, and PET CT is helpful for evaluating for distant spread. The primary tumor may appear as a focal mass, an ulcerated mass, or as a diffusely infiltrative process involving the gastric wall. Diffusely infiltrative tumors may be desmoplastic, stiffening the gastric wall that results in the linitis plastic pattern. Irregularity of the outer gastric contour, extension into the perigastric fat, and adjacent organ invasion can indicate the extent of local disease. CT is also used for the assessment of lymph node involvement, hematogenous spread to the liver, and direct seeding of the peritoneum with tumor involvement of the pelvis and ovaries.

Management

Early gastric adenocarcinoma may be treated with endoscopic resection; advanced disease requires surgical resection.

Further Reading

1. Fishman EK, Urban BA, Hruban RH. CT of the stomach: spectrum of disease. *RadioGraphics*. 1996; *16*(5): 1035–1054.

History

▶ 57-year-old man with persistent epigastric pain and dyspepsia.

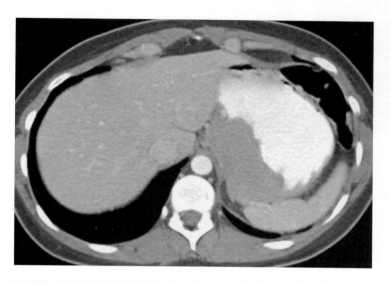

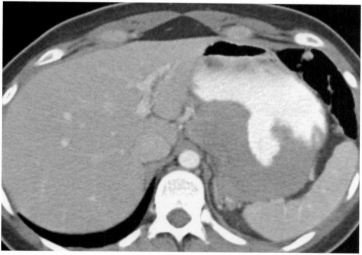

Case 27 Primary Gastric Lymphoma

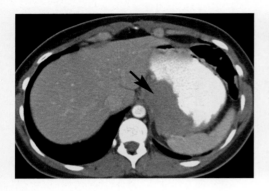 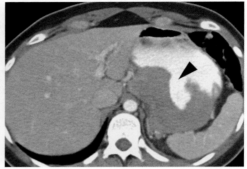

Findings

CT shows marked wall thickening of the gastric fundus and body (arrow) with preservation of the perigastric fat. The infiltrated gastric wall shows homogeneous attenuation. A large central ulcer (arrowhead) is present in the mass.

Differential Diagnosis

► Gastric adenocarcinoma: wall thickening is usually less prominent and more heterogeneous in CT attenuation, and invasion of perigastric fat is more common. Perigastric and celiac lymph nodes may be present, but nodes usually do not extend below the level of the renal veins.

► Metastasis: melanoma, lung, and breast cancer are the most common primary tumors to metastasize to the stomach. Widespread metastatic disease is usually present in the setting of gastric metastases.

Teaching Points

The stomach is the most common site for primary gastrointestinal lymphoma. Gastric lymphomas usually present in the fifth decade of life and tend to affect men more than women; however, in the HIV population, patients are much younger at diagnosis. Fewer than five percent of gastric malignancies are primary gastric lymphomas; non-Hodgkin B-cell lymphomas are the most common subtypes. Low-grade mucosa-associated lymphoid tissue (MALT) and high-grade B-cell lymphoma are associated with *H. pylori* infection. Prognosis mainly depends on histological grade; five-year mortality is nearly twice as high for patients with high-grade disease. Gastric lymphomas usually arise in the distal two-thirds of the stomach and often cause bulky homogeneous thickening of the gastric wall without significant distortion of the rugal folds. Low attenuation and necrosis within lymphomas is uncommon and suggests highly aggressive histology. The degree of wall thickening and abdominal adenopathy in low-grade lymphoma is frequently less severe compared to that of high-grade gastric lymphoma.

Management

CT and PET CT are used for tumor staging. CT can also identify complications from tumor burden or from treatment such as perforation, obstruction, or fistula formation.

Further Reading

1. Ghai S, Pattison J, Ghai S, O'Malley ME, Khalili K, Stephens M. Primary gastrointestinal lymphoma: spectrum of imaging findings with pathologic correlation. *RadioGraphics*. 2007; *27*(5): 1371–1388.

History

▶ 67-year-old man with remote history of prior resection of superficial spreading skin melanoma now complains of dysphagia and hematemesis.

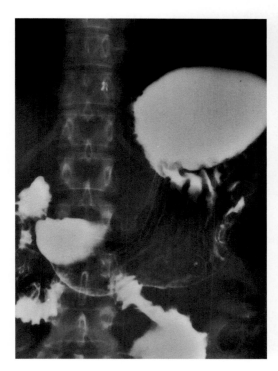 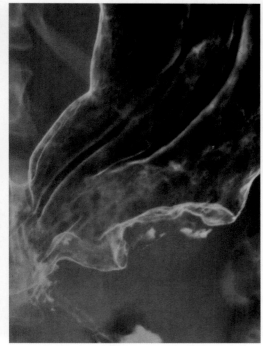

Case 28 Gastric Metastatic Melanoma

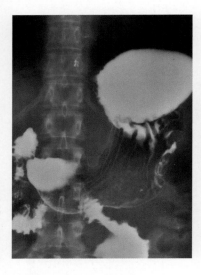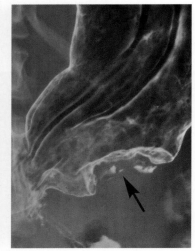

Findings

Upper gastrointestinal series shows a mass along the greater curvature of the stomach (arrow). Several irregular collections of barium along the mass correspond to ulcerations.

Differential Diagnosis

► Adenocarcinoma: may have an identical appearance.
► Gastrointestinal stromal tumor: large tumors that may ulcerate and may have a similar appearance.
► Lymphoma: usually causes extensive wall thickening and may ulcerate.
► Heterotopic pancreas: usually a small, well-defined, rounded or ovoid submucosal lesion along the antral portion of the greater curvature.
► Carcinoid: rare neoplasm that usually is less than 1 cm in size, multifocal, and associated with hypergastrinemia.

Teaching Points

Malignant melanoma is a common cutaneous malignancy associated with gastrointestinal tract metastases but may arise as a primary gastrointestinal primary tumor. Metastatic lesions are usually multiple in number, may be polypoid or infiltrative, and are often ulcerated. There is a very high incidence of gastrointestinal involvement in patients with primary cutaneous metastatic melanoma, with the stomach harboring disease in approximately 20 percent of patients; only the liver and small bowel are more often affected. More than half of patients with gastrointestinal involvement have metastatic disease of additional organ systems. Metastases may present at initial diagnosis or years later. The prognosis for metastatic disease carries an average survival rate of less than six months. Breast and lung primary tumors may also metastasize to the stomach.

Management

Most cutaneous melanoma metastases are 18-FDG avid at PET CT imaging. Given the high incidence of melanoma metastases to organs that are difficult to evaluate, such as bowel and muscle, PET CT should be considered for the determination of disease extent when metastases are suspected.

Further Reading

1. Liang KV, Sanderson SO, Nowakowski GS, Arora AS. Metastatic malignant melanoma of the gastrointestinal tract. *Mayo Clin Proc.* 2006; *81*(4): 511–516.

History

▶ 50-year-old woman with a history of hyperparathyroidism complains of abdominal pain, anorexia, and weight loss.

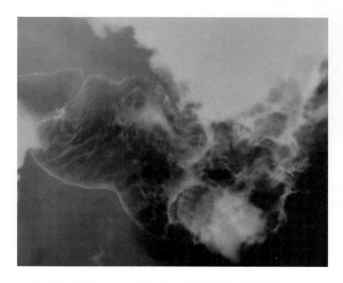

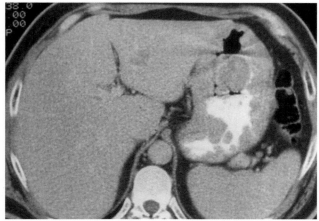

Case 29 Type 2 ECL-Cell Gastric Carcinoid

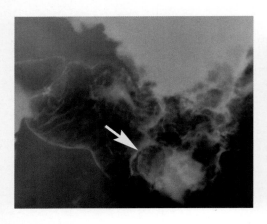 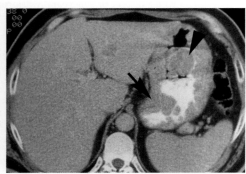

Findings

Upper gastrointestinal series (left) shows diffuse gastric fold thickening and a polypoid gastric mass (arrow) with a central ulcer. CT (right) shows a thickened and nodular gastric wall (arrow) and a 3.0 cm polypoid mass (arrowhead) in the gastric body that corresponds to the mass on the upper gastrointestinal series. The left lobe liver lesion was proven to be hemangioma.

Differential Diagnosis

- ▶ Multiple hyperplastic polyps: most common gastric polyp. Typically located in the gastric fundus and body, it is usually small, measuring less than 1.0 cm.
- ▶ Ménétrier disease: produces a hypertrophic gastritis characterized by thickened gastric folds but also has increased secretions and ulcerations.
- ▶ Lymphoma and gastric adenocarcinoma: may be considered in the differential diagnosis for extensive gastric wall thickening and a gastric mass.

Teaching Points

Gastric carcinoids are rare neoplasms that comprise less than 10 percent of all gastrointestinal carcinoids. Gastric carcinoids most often arise from enterochromaffin-like cells (ECL cells) of the fundus or body of the stomach. At least three subtypes are recognized. Type 1 carcinoids are the most common, usually found in older women, and are associated with autoimmune atrophic gastritis. Type 2 lesions are the least common and are found in patients with Zollinger-Ellison syndrome secondary to multiple endocrine neoplasia-1. Both type 1 and 2 carcinoids are usually less than 1 cm in size, multifocal, and associated with hypergastrinemia. Type 3 tumors are sporadic, occur more often in men, present as large solitary masses, and harbor a much worse prognosis than type 1 and 2 tumors.

Management

Prognostic factors for gastric carcinoids include tumor size, depth of invasion, lymph node involvement, and distant metastasis. The degree to which the tumors are under hormonal control is also of consideration. Type 1 and 2 carcinoids are usually treated conservatively with surveillance or polypectomy, and type 3 lesions require gastric resection.

Further Reading

1. Levy AD, Sobin LH. From the archives of the AFIP: Gastrointestinal carcinoids: imaging features with clinicopathologic comparison. *RadioGraphics*. 2007; *27*(1): 237–257.

History

▸ 64-year-old woman with lower abdominal pain.

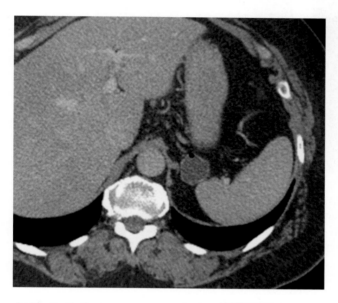

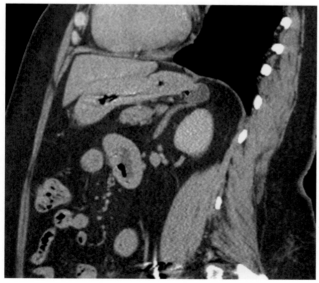

Case 30   Gastric Fundal Diverticulum

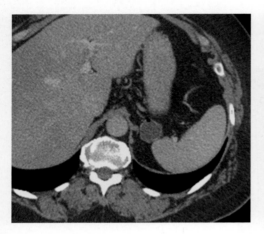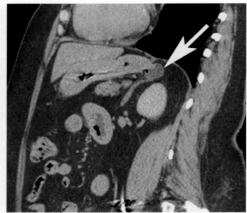

Findings

CT image (left) shows a small fluid-filled structure posterior to the stomach fundus without obvious involvement of other organs. A speck of gas is present in the nondependent portion of the collection. The collection (arrow) is inseparable from the stomach fundus on the sagittal view (right image).

Differential Diagnosis

► Adrenal mass: contiguity with the adrenal gland and absence of gas should be seen.
► Pancreatic pseudocyst: a history of pancreatitis or peripancreatic fat stranding is usually seen.
► Lymphadenopathy: will not be contiguous with the stomach. Does not contain gas or contrast.
► Accessory spleen: will enhance similar to the adjacent spleen.

Teaching Points

Gastric fundal diverticulum is a not uncommon finding at cross-sectional imaging and most typically occurs posterior to the stomach near the gastroesophageal junction and just below the left hemidiaphragm. When a gastric diverticulum contains gas or oral contrast, it does not pose a diagnostic dilemma. But when it is completely filled with fluid or intermediate-density material, it may be mistaken as lymphadenopathy or a cystic or solid mass at CT arising from the adrenal gland. Careful inspection of the adrenal gland will reveal non-contiguity of the structures.

Management

If a CT scan shows an ambiguous cystic structure in the left upper abdomen, the diagnosis of a gastric fundal diverticulum may be confirmed by comparison with prior imaging scans, repeat CT imaging with oral contrast material, or with an upper GI fluoroscopic study. These diverticula are rarely symptomatic, and no further work-up is generally required. Large or symptomatic diverticula may require surgical excision, which may be performed laparoscopically.

Further Readings

1. Gokan T, Ohgiya Y, Nobusawa H, Munechika H. Commonly encountered adrenal pseudotumours on CT. *Br J Radiol*. 2005; *78*(926): 170–174.
2. Tebala GD, Camperchioli I, Tognoni V, Innocenti P, Gaspari AL. Laparoscopic treatment of a gastric diverticulum. *Eur Rev Med Pharmacol Sci*. 2010; *14*(2): 135–138.

History

▶ 45-year-old woman with a history of a paraesophageal hiatal hernia with acute epigastric pain and vomiting.

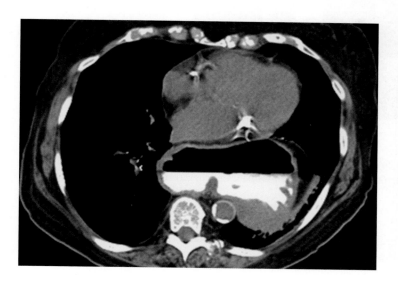

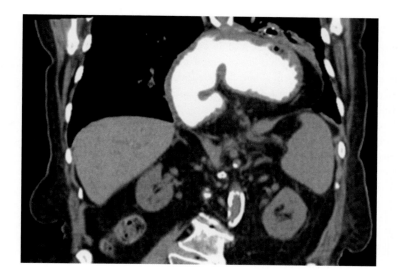

Case 31 Organoaxial Gastric Volvulus

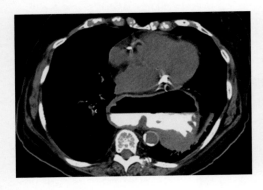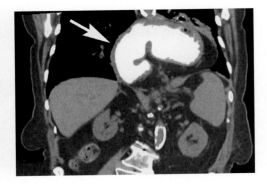

Findings

CT shows herniation of the stomach above the diaphragm and rotation of the stomach about its long axis, such that the greater curvature (arrow) is situated superior to the lesser curvature, consistent with organoaxial volvulus.

Differential Diagnosis

► Mesenteroaxial gastric volvulus: rotation occurs perpendicularly to the long axis of the stomach. Defects of the diaphragm are less common in this subtype.
► Paraesophageal hiatal hernia: paraesophageal hernias may be associated with organoaxial volvulus. In a pure paraesophageal hernia, the stomach herniates through the diaphragm alongside the esophagus, and the gastroesophageal junction remains in its normal position.

Teaching Points

Gastric volvulus is a rare condition with a peak incidence in the fifth decade of life; however, 20 percent of patients are less than one year old. Primary volvulus, which is less common, occurs below the diaphragm and is usually associated with neoplasia, adhesions, or ligament abnormalities. The secondary form occurs above the diaphragm and is often associated with a diaphragmatic defect. Organoaxial volvulus refers to rotation of the stomach around its longitudinal axis and is highly predisposed to strangulation. Mesenteroaxial volvulus, rotation about the short axis, is less common and more likely to occur in children. Organoaxial and mesenteroaxial volvulus may also occur together in the same clinical setting. In any case, rotation greater than 180 degrees generally results in gastric obstruction. Acute and chronic forms of volvulus are differentiated by speed of onset and degree of obstruction.

Management

Acute gastric volvulus is a surgical emergency due to the high risk of gastric wall perforation, vascular compromise, and necrosis. Mortality rates for acute volvulus range from 30 to 50 percent. In patients with chronic gastric volvulus, conservative medical management is less optimal secondary to the risk of future strangulation, and therefore these patients should be offered surgical correction.

Further Reading

1. Peterson CM, Anderson JS, Hara AK, Carenza JW, Menias CO. Volvulus of the gastrointestinal tract: Appearances at multimodality imaging. *RadioGraphics* 2009; *29*(5): 1281–1293.

Part 3   Duodenum

History

▶ 45-year-old man complains of solid and liquid dysphagia. He describes feeling food stick in the mid chest.

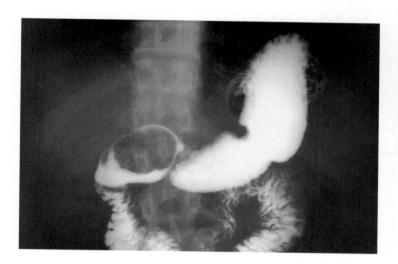

Case 32 Brunner Gland Hamartoma

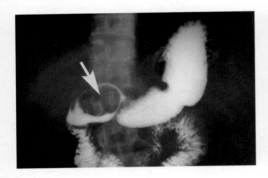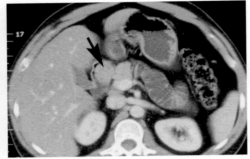

Findings

Barium examination of the stomach and duodenum shows a well-defined intraluminal polyp (arrow in left image) in the duodenal bulb. The polyp expands the bulb, but does not obstruct. Intravenous contrast-enhanced CT scan from a different patient with the same abnormality shows an enhancing intraluminal polypoid mass in the duodenal bulb (arrow in right image).

Differential Diagnosis

► Adenoma and adenocarcinoma: more common in the second portion of the duodenum in the periampullary region.
► Lymphoma: primary duodenal lymphoma is rare. Lymphoma more commonly involves the duodenum from adjacent peripancreatic and retroperitoneal lymph node enlargement.
► Gastrointestinal stromal tumor (GIST): tends to have central necrosis or hemorrhage as the tumor enlarges.
► Carcinoid: uncommon in the duodenum, may be solitary or multifocal small intramural or polypoid lesions.
► Pancreatic heterotopia: may have central umbilication or ulceration.

Teaching Points

Brunner gland hamartoma most commonly arises in the first or second portion of the duodenum, where there is the largest concentration of Brunner glands. Although these are benign lesions, there have been reports of carcinomas arising within the lesions. The lesions may cause abdominal pain, duodenal obstruction, intussusception, and obstruction of the common bile duct or pancreatic duct. Patients may be asymptomatic with incidental discovery of the lesions. On barium studies, these lesions may be sessile or pedunculated, but they generally are smoothly marginated and oval or round in shape. On CT, they may have homogeneous or heterogeneous enhancement following intravenous contrast administration.

Management

Endoscopic polypectomy or limited surgical excision is the treatment of choice for symptomatic lesions.

Further Reading
1. Patel ND, Levy AD, Mehrotra AK and Sobin LH. Brunner's gland hyperplasia and hamartoma: imaging features with clinicopathologic correlation. *Am J Roentgenol. 2006; 187*: 715–722.

History

▶ 55-year-old man with epigastric pain, jaundice, and recent weight loss.

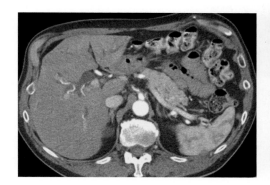
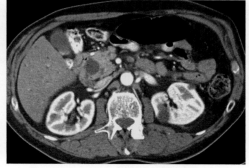
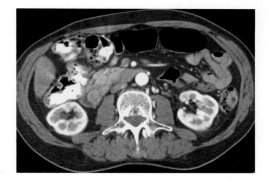

Case 33 Duodenal Periampullary Adenocarcinoma

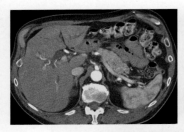
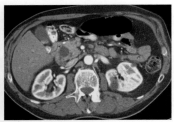
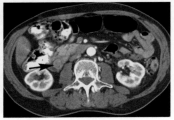

Findings

CT images show intra- and extrahepatic bile duct dilatation. An enhancing mass arises from the periampullary duodenal mucosa (arrow, bottom image).

Differential Diagnosis

► Pancreatic adenocarcinoma and ampullary adenocarcinoma: may be indistinguishable from periampullary duodenal tumors. A lesion centered in the distal common bile duct or pancreas suggests the tumor arises from these locations.
► Carcinoid tumors and endocrine carcinomas: typically enhance more intensely than adenocarcinomas following contrast administration.
► Somatostatin producing carcinoid tumors (somatostainomas): occur in patients with neurofibromatosis type 1 (NF-1), and occur exclusively in the periampullary region.

Teaching Points

Periampullary duodenal adenocarcinomas arise from the periampullary duodenal mucosa, which is the most common site for small bowel adenocarcinomas. They may arise de novo or from pre-existing adenomas or villous adenomas. Patients may present with nonspecific symptoms such as anemia, malaise, epigastric pain, and/or weight loss. Biliary and pancreatic ductal obstruction may occur even when tumors are small, and can cause jaundice, cholangitis, or pancreatitis. Periampullary duodenal adenocarcinomas may manifest as intraluminal polypoid masses, ulcerated masses, or infiltrating masses in the region of the duodenal papilla. Infiltrating lesions may invade the pancreas and distal common bile duct, becoming indistinguishable from pancreatic and ampullary carcinomas. The finding of a periampullary mucosal lesion is a supportive finding of the tumor originating from the periampullary duodenal mucosa.

Management

Periampullary duodenal adenocarcinomas are staged according to the TNM system, and resectable lesions should be completely excised with wide margins. The standard operation is a pancreaticoduodenectomy.

Further Readings

1. Buck JL, Elsayed AM. Ampullary tumors: radiologic-pathologic correlation. *RadioGraphics*. 1993; *13*(1): 193–212.
2. Yeo CJ, Sohn TA, Cameron JL, et al. Periampullary adenocarcinoma: analysis of 5-year survivors. *Ann Surg*. 1998; *227*(6): 821–831.

History

▶ 30-year-old man with right upper quadrant pain.

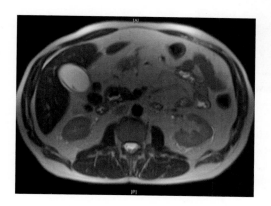

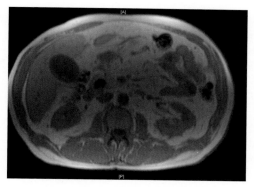

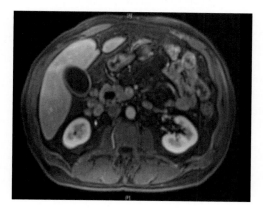

Case 34 Peri-Ampullary (Juxta-Papillary) Diverticulum

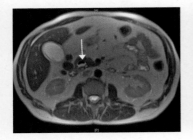 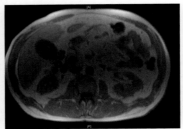 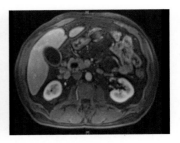

Findings

Axial T2-weighted image (left) shows a cystic focus (arrow) in the head of the pancreas, with bright signal consistent with fluid and nondependent dark signal suggestive of air. The in-phase T1-weighted image (center) shows susceptability artifact that confirms the presence of air. Following IV gadolinium (right), there is no enhancement within this lesion. There is no associated common bile duct (CBD) or pancreatic duct dilation.

Differential Diagnosis

▶ Pseudocyst: occurs as a sequela of pancreatitis. It is well circumscribed and fluid attenuation but may contain internal debris. It does not communicate with the main pancreatic duct.

▶ Cystic neoplasm: such as intraductal papillary mucinous neoplasm which communicates with the main pancreatic duct, mucinous cystic neoplasm, and serous microcystic pancreatic adenoma. These lesions do not contain air.

Teaching Points

Peri-ampullary/juxta-papillary duodenal diverticula have an incidence in the adult population of 5 to 10 percent, are generally asymptomatic, and usually detected incidentally. They arise from the medial wall of the second portion of the duodenum 2 to 2.5 cm from the ampulla of Vater. They can make cannulation of the ampulla difficult during ERCP.

Duodenal diverticula may contain fluid which creates a bright signal on T2-weighted images, or can contain gas-containing debris which causes a blooming/susceptibility artifact on gradient echo in-phase sequences. Blooming artifact refers to decrease in signal in and immediately around an focus that contains gas or ferromagnetic material due to magnetic field inhomogeneity that occurs in sequences with longer TE's. It is difficult to differentiate diverticula from a cystic pancreatic lesion if no gas is present. In unusual cases, large diverticula may affect the function of the ampulla of Vater and distal common bile duct

(CBD), and can cause jaundice, primary choledocholithiasis, or cholangitis. Debris impaction in a diverticulum also may cause diverticulitis. Severe diverticular hemorrhage may occur.

Management

Usually peri-ampullary/juxta-papillary duodenal diverticula are asymptomatic, and they can generally be ignored. They may be surgically resected if they hemorrhage or develop refractory diverticulitis.

Further Readings

1. Perdikakis E, Chryssou EG, Karantanas A. Diagnosis of peri-ampullary duodenal diverticula: the value of new imaging techniques. *Annals of Gastroenterology.* 2011; *24*: 192–199.
2. Tsitouridis I, Emmanouilidou M, Goutsaridou F, et al. MRCP in the evaluation of patients with duodenal peri-ampullary diverticulum. *European Journal of Radiology.* 2003; *47*: 154–160.

History

▶ 39-year-old man complains of abdominal pain.

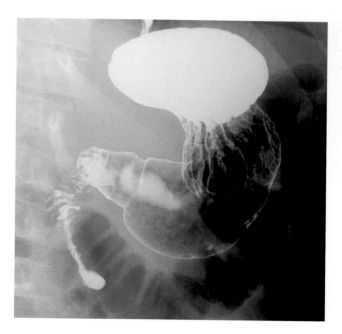

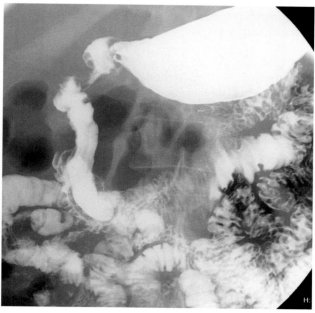

Case 35 Intraluminal Duodenal Diverticulum

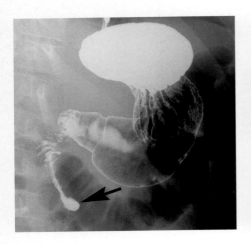 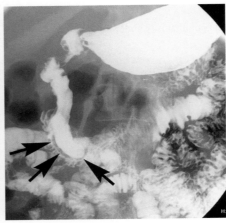

Findings

Upper gastrointestinal series shows barium filling a blind-ending, oval-shaped sac within the duodenal lumen (arrow in left image). Later in the exam (right image), the sac is surrounded by a radiolucent line (arrows in right image) and barium.

Differential Diagnosis

- Duplication cyst: may be located within the duodenal wall and may communicate with the lumen so that the cyst fills with barium. Duplication cysts have a smooth contour and usually exert mass effect to narrow the duodenal lumen as they enlarge with fluid or fill with barium.
- Acquired duodenal diverticula: common in the periampullary region of the duodenum along the medial aspect of the duodenum. They may have a wide or narrow neck and project extraluminally.

Teaching Points

Intraluminal duodenal diverticula are rare, congenital intraluminal webs or mucosal diaphragms that elongate intraluminally over time due to peristalsis and the forward propulsion of food. An intraluminal duodenal diverticulum usually originates in the second portion of the duodenum near the ampulla of Vater. It may contain a fenestration or opening at its tip or along the course of the diverticulum. Its appearance on barium exams is often called the *windsock sign*. The radiolucent rim formed by barium both outside and within the diverticulum has been called the *halo sign*. The abnormality may present in childhood or early adulthood with nausea, vomiting, or epigastric pain. The diverticulum may intermittently obstruct the ampulla of Vater, causing pancreatitis and biliary obstruction. Patients with intraluminal duodenal diverticula are reported to have a 40 percent prevalence of coexisting congenital anomalies such as Hirschsprung disease, choledochocele, annular pancreas, congenital heart disease, omphalocele, situs inversus, portal vein anomalies, malrotation, Ladd bands, Down syndrome, bladder exstrophy, and renal hypoplasia.

Management

Duodenotomy with surgical excision or endoscopic excision is necessary to prevent complications such as duodenal obstruction, stasis, impaction of food, pancreatitis, or biliary obstruction.

Further Readings

1. Takamatsu S, Gabata T, Matsui O, Noto M, Ninomiya I, Nonomura A. Intraluminal duodenal diverticulum: MR findings. *Abdom Imaging*. 2006; *31*(1): 39–42.
2. Materne R. The duodenal wind sock sign. *Radiology*. 2001; *218*(3): 749–750.

History

▶ 19-year-old woman complains of abdominal pain.

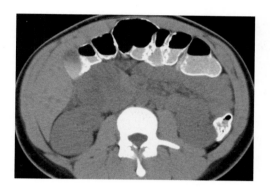

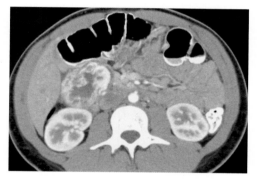

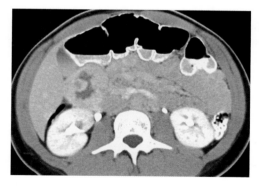

Case 36 Duodenal Gastrointestinal Stromal Tumor

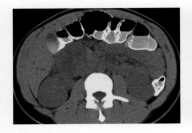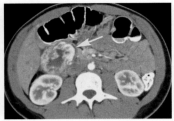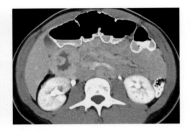

Findings

CT images show a mass between the head of the pancreas and right lobe of the liver. The mass (arrow) compresses the duodenum and displaces it to the right. The mass has heterogeneous peripheral enhancement with central hypoattenuation.

Differential Diagnosis

▶ Adenocarcinoma: the periampullary region is the most common location for duodenal adenocarcinoma, but tumors are usually hypovascular.
▶ Lymphoma: duodenal involvement is usually secondary to peripancreatic and retroperitoneal lymph nodes. The majority of lymphomas are homogeneous in CT attenuation.
▶ Metastatic disease: retroperitoneal or peripancreatic lymph nodes may mimic a duodenal mass.

Teaching Points

Gastrointestinal stromal tumor (GIST) is the most common mesenchymal neoplasm of the gastrointestinal tract. Most commonly occurring in the stomach, 20 to 30 percent of GISTs arise in the small bowel. Clinical symptomatology depends upon size and location. Gastrointestinal bleeding is common when the mass ulcerates. Though submucosal in location, GISTs may have intraluminal and/or exoenteric extension. The margins of the mass are usually well defined, but ulceration and irregularity may be seen on the luminal side of the mass. On CT, central hypoattenuation may represent intratumoral necrosis, degeneration, or hemorrhage. The enhancing portions of the mass are typically heterogeneous. Calcification and cavitation may also occur. Adjacent lymphadenopathy is typically absent. When lymphadenopathy is present, other neoplasm, such as adenocarcinoma should be favored. GISTs metastasize hematogenously to the liver, followed by distant sites and to the peritoneal cavity.

Management

Surgical resection of the primary lesion is the conventional treatment for GISTs. Pathologically, tumor size and mitotic rate are used to assess malignant potential; c-kit-inhibitors are used to treat recurrent and metastatic GIST.

Further Readings

1. Levy AD, Remotti HE, et al. From the Archives of AFIP: Gastrointestinal stromal tumors: Radiologic features with Pathologic Correlation. *RadioGraphics*. 2003; *23*: 283–304.
2. Kim HC, Lee JM, Son KR, et al. Gastrointestinal stromal tumors of the duodenum: CT and barium study findings. *Am J Roentgenol*. 2004; *183*(2): 415–419.

History

▸ 45-year-old man with abdominal pain after a motor vehicle accident.

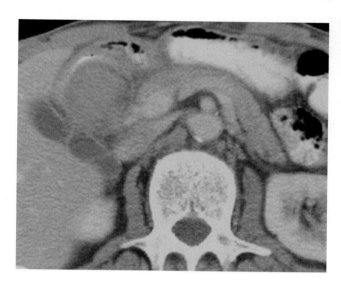

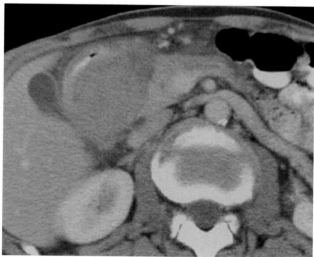

Case 37 Duodenal Hematoma

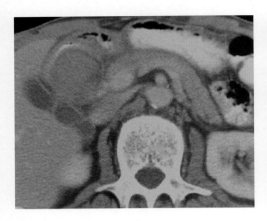 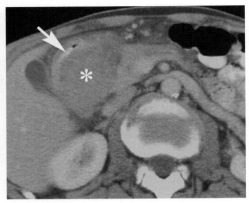

Findings

CT shows a high attenuation mass expanding the duodenal wall (asterisk) and deviating the duodenal lumen (arrow) to the right. The adjacent pancreas is normal. There is no extraluminal air or contrast.

Differential Diagnosis

► Gastrointestinal stromal tumors (GISTs): in the absence of trauma, should be considered in the differential diagnosis of an intramural mass of the duodenum. Small GISTs may have homogeneous enhancement, but larger GISTs tend to be more heterogeneous and may cavitate.

► Duplication cyst: tend to contain low attenuation fluid, but may have higher attenuation fluid if they contain proteinaceous debris or hemorrhage.

► Abscess: inflammatory fat stranding, fluid, and extraluminal air from a perforated ulcer diverticulum.

Teaching Points

Classically, duodenal hematomas occur as the result of a seat belt injury, which causes anterior to posterior compression of the duodenum on the spine, in rapid deceleration motor vehicle accidents. Other forms of blunt abdominal trauma may cause similar injuries. Duodenal hematomas should be distinguished from duodenal perforation and disruption. Duodenal perforation is suspected when there is discontinuity in the duodenal wall or extraluminal oral contrast or gas. Duodenal contusions with hematoma formation may cause focal wall thickening or an intramural mass from the hematoma. In the acute setting, the hematoma may have high CT attenuation from acute blood. Over time, the hematoma will have mixed attenuation or fluid attenuation. Fluid and fat stranding may also be present in the anterior perirenal space of the retroperitoneum. It is important to closely inspect the adjacent organs such as the pancreas, gallbladder, liver, and spleen as well as the vasculature for additional sites of injury.

Management

Duodenal hematomas without perforation are usually managed conservatively. Perforation and rupture frequently require operative repair. The extent of injury, status of the vasculature, and presence of associated pancreatic injury in context with the patient's clinical status is used to determine management.

Further Reading

1. Linsenmaier U, Wirth S, Reiser M, Korner M. Diagnosis and classification of pancreatic and duodenal injuries in emergency radiology. *RadioGraphics*. 2008; *28*(6): 1591–1602.

History

▶ 52-year-old man with severe abdominal pain and a remote past history of peptic ulcer disease.

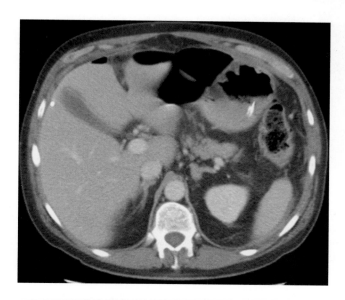

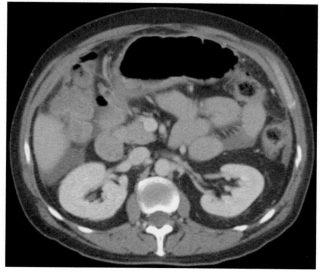

Case 38 Perforated Duodenal Ulcer

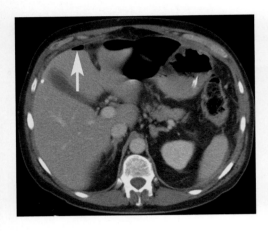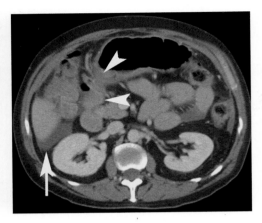

Findings

CT (left) shows free intraperitoneal air (arrow) by the falciform ligament, in the left anterior subphrenic space and between the left lobe of the liver and gastric body in the left anterior subhepatic space. A more inferior image (right) shows trace fluid in Morison pouch and along the liver tip (arrow) with wall thickening and fat stranding of the gastric antrum and duodenal bulb (arrowheads).

Differential Diagnosis

► Perforated appendicitis or diverticulitis: uncommon to see free air in the left anterior subphrenic space. Bowel wall thickening, fat stranding, and fluid with pockets of extraluminal air are typically concentrated in the lower abdomen or pelvis.

► Perforated small bowel diverticulum: may show findings similar to perforated peptic ulcer disease. The fat stranding and bowel wall thickening centers on the diverticulum.

Teaching Points

Despite the decreased incidence of peptic ulcer disease because of improved prevention and treatment, perforated ulcers remain a serious life-threatening complication. CT is more sensitive than abdominal radiographs for identification of pneumoperitoneum. The site of perforation can be suggested based on several observations: the distribution of intraperitoneal air, the presence of fluid and fat stranding, and the location of fat stranding and thickening of the affected bowel. The "CT falciform ligament sign" refers to air or fluid in the left anterior subphrenic space surrounding the falciform ligament. When this sign is present, perforations are usually in the stomach or small bowel. In general, when large quantities of free intraperitoneal air are present in the absence of instrumentation, the most common source of the free air is a gastric or duodenal ulcer perforation.

Management

Most patients with perforated peptic ulcer will need emergency surgery such as a patch repair or resection.

Further Readings

1. Yeung K, Chang M, Hsiao C, Huang J. CT evaluation of gastrointestinal tract perforation. *Journal of Clinical Imaging*. 2004; *28*: 329–333.
2. Chen CH, Huang HS, Yang CC, Hey YH. The features of perforated peptic ulcers in conventional computed tomography. *Hepatogastroenterology*. 2001 Sep–Oct; *48*(41): 1393–1396.

Part 4

Small Intestine

History

▶ 32-year-old woman with chronic abdominal pain.

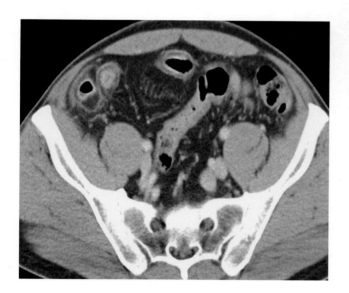

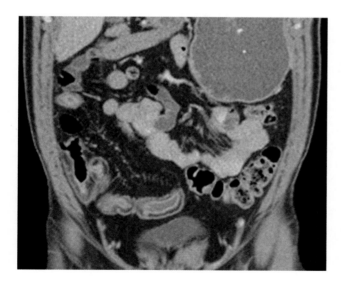

Case 39 Crohn Disease with Fibrofatty Proliferation

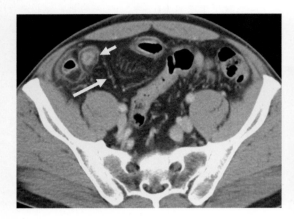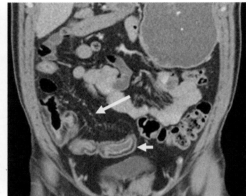

Findings

Axial (left) and coronal (right) CT images show abnormally thickened ileal bowel segments with mural stratification from mucosal and muscular hyperenhancement sandwiching a layer of hypodense submucosal fat (short arrow) and edema. The mesenteric fat is asymmetrically expanded, displaces bowel loops, and encases engorged peri-enteric vessels, which are also known as the vasa recti (long arrow).

Differential Diagnosis

► Infectious enteritis: imaging findings typically reflect acute inflammation such as mucosal hyperenhancement. The chronic changes seen here would be unusual.

► Graft versus host disease: appearance and distribution of the abnormalities may be identical, but the patient should have a history of allogenic stem cell transplantation.

► Radiation enteritis: early stages may show inflamed bowel within the distribution of the irradiated field that may produce strictures. The patient would have a history of radiation therapy.

Teaching Points

Crohn disease is a chronic inflammatory disorder typified by transmural inflammation and multifocality that may involve the alimentary tract at any level, but has a predilection for the terminal ileum and colon. Imaging helps establish the diagnosis and characterize disease extent, severity, and complications. Active inflammation is characterized by mucosal and muscular hyperenhancement, a thickened, edematous bowel wall, and engorged vasa recta. It is important to recognize complications such as sinus tracts, fistulas, and abscesses, as well as any luminal narrowing with pre-stenotic dilatation that indicates small bowel strictures. The latter may develop from mural fibrosis or mural edema in the setting of active disease. Submucosal fat deposition and proliferation of mesenteric fat, so called "creeping fat" or "fibrofatty proliferation," may be associated with chronically involved segments of small bowel.

Management

Disease distribution and the presence or absence of mesenteric complications should be reported in order to guide medical (antibiotic and immunosuppressive) and surgical therapy. It is useful to note the location and length of each strictured segment as well as the presence of sinus tracts and abscesses for the purpose of interventional and surgical planning.

Further Reading

1. Hara A, Swartz PG. CT enterography of Crohn disease. *Abdominal Imaging*. 2009; *34*: 289–295.

History

▶ 67-year-old man with history of chronic abdominal pain and diarrhea presents with acute pain and bloating.

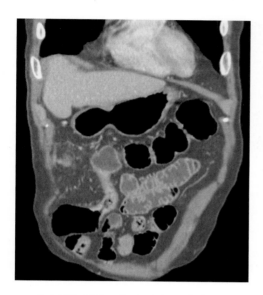

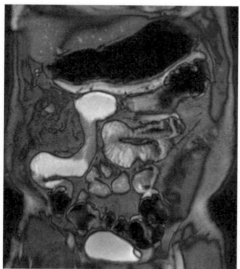

Case 40 Crohn Disease with Stricture

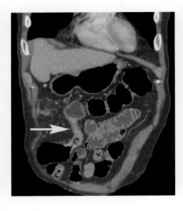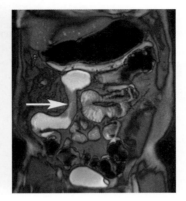

Findings

CT (left) shows focal ileal wall thickening, narrowing, and hyperenhancement (arrow) and adjacent fibrofatty proliferation. MR enterography (right image) two years later shows persistent ileal mural thickening and stricturing (arrow).

Differential Diagnosis

► Small bowel lymphoma: usually more nodular or concentric bowel mass with associated lymphadenopathy. Aneurysmal dilation of involved bowel segment can be seen.

► Small bowel adenocarcinoma: uncommon and may present as polypoid mass or irregular "apple-core" lesion, usually in the duodenum or jejunum, and may be associated with inflammatory enteritis.

► Ischemic enteritis: presents acutely with segmental bowel wall thickening and possible pneumatosis or mural nonenhancement, occasionally with superior mesenteric artery or vein thrombus.

► Infectious enteritis: other pathogens that characteristically involve the distal ileum and cause stricturing such as Tuberculosis may have a similar appearance.

► Graft-versus-host disease: history of bone marrow transplant is necessary for the diagnosis.

Teaching Points

Crohn disease is a chronic, transmural inflammatory process that can occur in any segment of bowel, but most commonly affects the terminal ileum. The prevalence is approximately 7 per 100,000 persons and is increasing. The age of onset is bimodal, with the first peak occurring at ages 15 to 30 and a smaller second peak at ages 60 to 80. Evaluation for acute inflammation and complications is increasingly performed with CT or MR enterography. Characteristic imaging findings include discontinuous segments of bowel wall thickening, mucosal or mural hyperenhancement leading to a "stratified" appearance that shows inner mucosal hyperenhancement and hypoattenuation of the adjacent, edematous submucosa. Adjacent mesenteric changes such as fibrofatty proliferation, lymphadenopathy and mesenteric hypervascularity (known as the comb sign because of its appearance in imaging) are often present. Common complications include mesenteric abscesses, strictures or fistulas/sinus tracts.

Management

Medical management may involve anti-inflammatory medications (mesalamine, sulfasalazine), steroids, and/or immunosuppressants. Stricturing of involved segments may occur, even after successful treatment of acute flares. Resection of diseased segments of bowel and fistulae may be undertaken, but recurrent disease is common.

Further Reading

1. Lee SS, Kim AY, Yang SK, Chung JW, Kim SY, Park SH, Ha HK. Crohn Disease of the Small Bowel: Comparison of CT Enterography, MR Enterography, and Small-Bowel Follow-Through as Diagnostic Techniques. *Radiology*. 2009; *251*: 751–761.

History

▶ 33-year-old female with abdominal pain and weight loss.

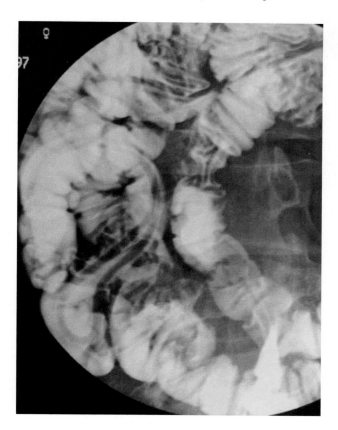

Case 41 Ascariasis

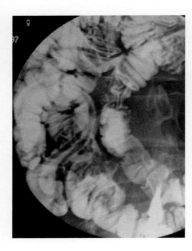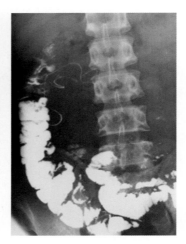

Findings

Single spot fluoroscopic image from a barium follow-through study shows an 8 to 10 cm linear worm-like filling defect in the region of the distal ileum. Delayed small bowel follow-through radiograph from another patient shows thin, linear collections of barium (arrow) in the intestinal tract of the worm.

Differential Diagnosis

▶ *Taenia solium* or *T. saginata*: these tapeworms are identified as thin, linear or double lines of radiolucencies on barium examinations. Unlike *Ascaris* roundworms, *Taenia* do not ingest the barium.

▶ *Trichuris trichiura*: roundworm that inhabits the colon, attaching to and superficially invading the mucosa. It appears as a ring-shaped lucency in the colon on barium examinations.

Teaching Points

Ascaris lumbricoides is a roundworm that inhabits the small bowel of approximately one-fourth of the world's population. Adult worms grow to as much as 35 cm in length and may live 6 to 12 months. They are transmitted via the fecal-oral route. Most people are asymptomatic but can present with vague abdominal pain, nausea, vomiting, nutritional deficiency, or a history of passing worms orally or rectally. Complications of ascariasis include mechanical small bowel obstruction, volvulus, or intussusception. The worms may penetrate the intestinal mucosa and migrate to the lungs, where they can cause bronchopneumonia. They can also lodge in the pancreaticobiliary ductal system, causing pancreatitis, cholecystitis, or liver abscess.

On barium studies, an *Ascaris* is an elongated, worm-like filling defect in the small bowel. Two worms seen side by side look like tram-tracks. On delayed images, barium ingested by the worm may highlight the worm's slender intestinal tract. On ultrasound, worms are hypoechoic, occasionally writhing tubular structures with echogenic walls, with the digestive tract of the worm forming two similar echogenic lines. CT is helpful in confirming complications associated with infestation.

Management

Stool samples are diagnostic for ascariasis, which is treated with albendazole. Surgery may be necessary to treat complications.

Further Reading

1. Ortega C, Ogawa N, Rocha M, et al. Helminthic diseases in the abdomen: an epidemiologic and radiological overview. *Radiographics.* 2010; *30*: 253–267.

History

▶ 35-year-old man with AIDS presents with right lower quadrant abdominal pain and intermittent fever.

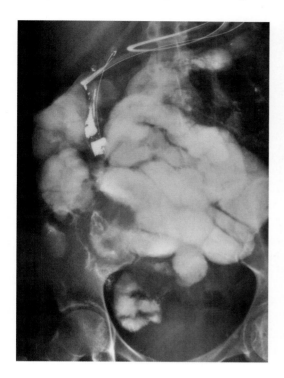
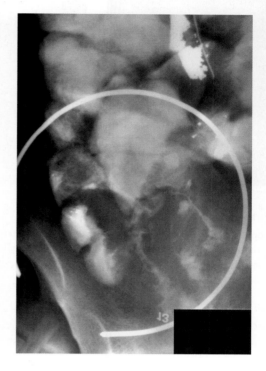

Case 42   Ileocolic Tuberculosis

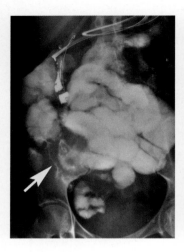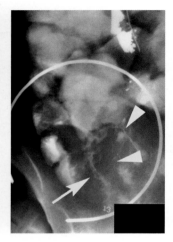

Findings

Supine abdominal radiograph and spot film from a barium small bowel follow through shows a long segment stricture of the terminal ileum (arrows) and multiple fistulous tracts (arrowheads) extending from the terminal ileum to adjacent ileal segments. Dilated small bowel proximal to the ileum suggests partial small bowel obstruction. The cecal tip is deformed.

Differential Diagnosis

- ▶ Crohn disease: may be indistinguishable from tuberculosis on barium studies. Cecal contraction and narrowing is usually more extensive in tuberculosis than in Crohn disease.
- ▶ Lymphoma: has more smooth mass effect and fewer associated mucosal changes such as ulceration, nodularity.
- ▶ Adenocarcinoma: may form fistula to adjacent segments of bowel if perforation occurs. There is typically mass effect from infiltration of the tumor in the wall or a polypoid lesion.
- ▶ Amebiasis: cecal and ascending colonic wall thickening, ulceration, and nodularity. The terminal ileum is usually spared.

Teaching Points

Gastrointestinal tuberculosis is uncommon in developed countries, occurring predominantly in the AIDS population, other immunosuppressed populations, and recent immigrants from countries where tuberculosis continues to be endemic. The ileocecal region is the most common site of gastrointestinal involvement because of the extensive lymphatics in the region. Tuberculosis causes mucosal ulcerations of varying size in the terminal ileum and cecum. There may be nodularity of the adjacent mucosa. Over time, extensive retraction and scarring may result in stricture formation. The ulcers may extend beyond the bowel to form sinus tracts and fistula to adjacent segments of bowel. The cecum may become contracted with a patulous ileocecal valve.

Management

Ileocecal tuberculosis is managed with a combination of medical and surgical therapy. Surgical approaches are used for complications such as bowel obstruction and fistula repair.

Further Readings

1. Brown JH, Berman JJ, Blickman JG, Chew FS. Primary ileocecal tuberculosis. *Am J Roentgenol.* 1993; *160*(2): 278.
2. Engin G, Balk E. Imaging findings of intestinal tuberculosis. *J Comput Assist Tomogr.* 2005; *29*(1): 37–41.

History

▶ 61-year-old man with severe osteoarthritis, intermittent nausea, vomiting, and abdominal distension and pain.

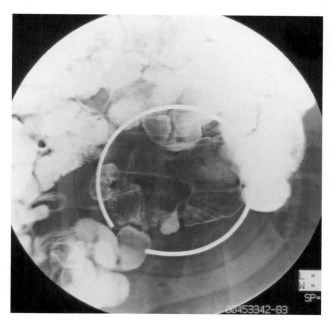

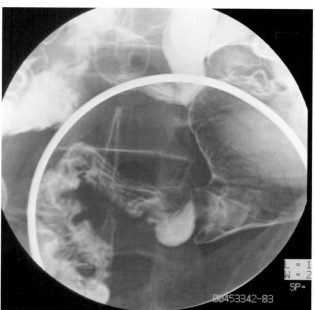

Case 43 NSAID Stricture

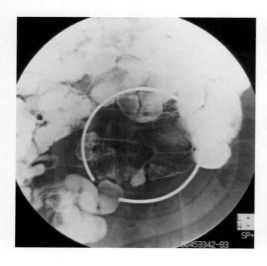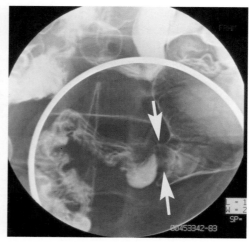

Findings

Image from a small bowel follow through exam shows a short, smoothly marginated stricture (arrows) in the ileum. There is no associated mass effect. There is pre-stenotic dilatation of the ileum proximal to the stricture.

Differential Diagnosis

▶ Crohn disease: strictures are common in the fibrostenotic phase of Crohn disease. Stricture length and number are highly variable. Skip lesions, fistulas, and other features of advanced Crohn disease may be present.

▶ Tuberculosis: ascending colon and cecum are more commonly involved.

▶ Radiation enteropathy: strictures may form as sequela of radiation enteritis and involve the irradiated bowel.

▶ Post-traumatic or post-surgical strictures: strictures may occur at sites of prior fistulas, hematomas, or small bowel repairs.

Teaching Points

Nonsteroidal anti-inflammatory drug (NSAID) injury to the small bowel is increasingly recognized as a complication in patients who take NSAIDs. Erosions, ulcers, and diaphragm-like strictures characterize NSAID injury. Ulcers are punctate, linear, and circumferential. Strictures form from chronic inflammation and fibrosis. They are classically web- or diaphragm-like, measuring 2 to 5 mm in thickness. Those patients with strictures have obstructive symptoms. The ileum is the most commonly affected location in the small bowel. A high index of suspicion is necessary to make the diagnosis because the strictures are difficult to identify on conventional small bowel follow through and usually are not seen on CT. The pathogenesis of the small bowel injury is not fully understood. Patients with NSAID injury to the small bowel frequently have anemia and occult gastrointestinal bleeding.

Management

NSAIDs should be discontinued in patients with all forms of NSAID enteropathy. Surgical resection of the diaphragm-like stricture is necessary to alleviate partial or complete small bowel obstructions.

Further Reading

1. Allison MC, Howatson AG, Torrance CJ, Lee FD, Russell RI. Gastrointestinal damage associated with the use of nonsteroidal antiinflammatory drugs. *N Engl J Med.* 1992; *327*(11): 749–754.

History

▶ 43-year-old woman with abdominal pain and watery diarrhea.

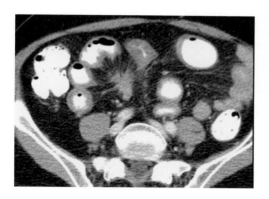

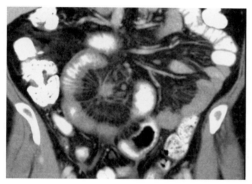

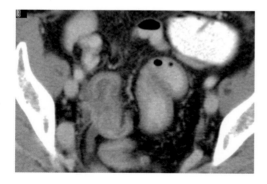

Case 44 Ileal Carcinoid

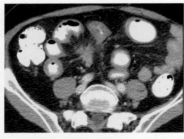
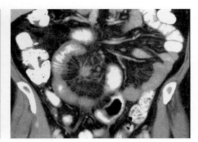
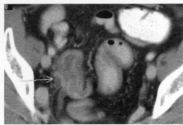

Findings

CT images show a spiculated mass within the mesentery (arrow). There is wall thickening and angulation of adjacent small bowel loops. Mesenteric lymph nodes are also present (arrowhead). There is a short segment of circumferential small bowel wall thickening (arrow on bottom image) with abnormal mucosal enhancement.

Differential Diagnosis

▶ Retractile mesenteritis: also known as sclerosing mesenteritis or mesenteric lipodystrophy, produces increased mesenteric attenuation. It does not encase vessels, but spares them with a lucent halo of fat surrounding the vessels.
▶ Lymphoma or metastasis: solitary or multiple masses in the mesentery.

Teaching Points

Ileal carcinoid arises from the submucosal APUD (amine precursor uptake and decarboxylation cells) cells of the ileum. It is a slow-growing lesion and most patients are asymptomatic. On imaging, the primary bowel lesion is rarely seen but may be apparent as an asymmetric or concentric region of mural bowel wall thickening with associated hyperenhancement. The metastatic deposit in the mesentery may be spiculated because the serotonin produced by the tumor incites a desmoplastic reaction. The mass may have fine stippled or coarse calcifications within it. The bowel may be retracted by the mesenteric metastasis and form a characteristic kink or hairpin turn. The localized production of serotonin may also cause strictures in the adjacent mesenteric vasculature that may cause ischemia. Patients may develop carcinoid syndrome, which occurs when vaso-active hormones are released into the systemic circulation, typically 5-HIAA (5-hydroxyindoleacetic acid) when the tumor has metastasized to the liver. This systemic syndrome causes symptoms such as flushing, bronchoconstriction, and diarrhea.

Management

Surgery is considered for primary resection of the tumor and the mesenteric mass. For liver metastases, resection versus chemoembolization can be considered. Systemic treatment is usually with the somatostatin analog octreotide.

Further Reading

1. Levy A, Sobin L. From the archives of the AFIP: Gastrointestinal carcinoids: imaging features with clinicopathological comparison. *RadioGraphics.* 2007; *27*: 237–257.

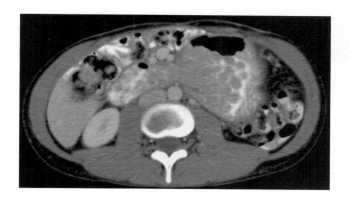

History

► 31-year-old man with gastrointestinal bleeding.

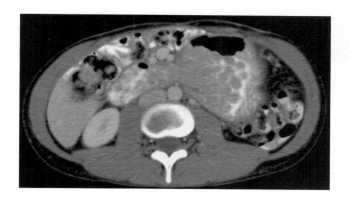

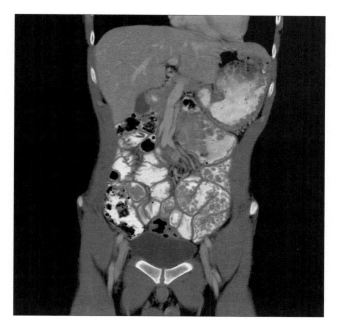

Case 45 Peutz-Jeghers Syndrome

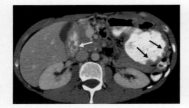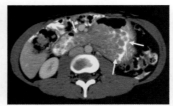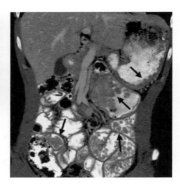

Findings

Axial (left image) and coronal (right image) contrast-enhanced CT images show innumerable gastric and small bowel polyps (arrows), most of which are smaller than 1 cm. A confluent collection of polyps is present in the third portion of the duodenum.

Differential Diagnosis

▶ Lymphoid hyperplasia: most commonly seen in children less than 2 years old or adults with late onset immunodeficiency syndrome. Typically, the bowel mucosa is studded with innumerable small uniform lesions (1 to 3 mm) that may have central umbilication.

▶ Familial adenomatous polyposis: numerous colonic polyps (anywhere from 500 to 2,500) carpet the colonic mucosa and involve the rectum.

▶ Juvenile polyposis: rarely occurs in the small bowel. Rectosigmoid involvement occurs in 80 percent of patients.

▶ Cronkhite-Canada syndrome: later age of presentation (42 to 75 years) with distinct clinical features (diarrhea, alopecia, nail atrophy).

Teaching Points

Peutz-Jeghers syndrome is a rare autosomal dominant disorder characterized by intestinal polyposis and mucocutaneous pigmentation. It is the most frequent polyposis syndrome to involve the small intestine. The jejunum and ileum are more commonly affected than the duodenum. Although polyps most commonly arise in the small intestine they may occur anywhere from the stomach to the rectum. The average age of presentation is 25 years, with males and females affected equally. Patients can present with intermittent abdominal pain due to small bowel intussusception caused by polyps or rectal bleeding and chronic anemia from polyp ulceration. Histologically, these polyps are hamartomatous and benign. However, foci of dysplasia, which may progress to malignancy, may occur within the polyps. Larger polyps tend to have a multilobulated surface while smaller ones (1 to 2 mm) may be smoother and sessile.

Management

Patients have an increased risk of developing gastrointestinal adenocarcinomas with the mean age at diagnosis being 40 years. The majority of cancers occur in the stomach, duodenum, and colon. There is also an increased risk of extraintestinal malignancies (pancreas, breast, pelvic, testicular, ovary). Because of this increased risk, cancer surveillance is recommended.

Further Reading

1. Rufener SL, Koujok K, McKenna BJ, et al. Small bowel intussuseption secondary to Peutz-Jeghers polyp. *RadioGraphics*. 2008; *28*: 284–288.

History

▶ 75-year-old man complains of abdominal pain.

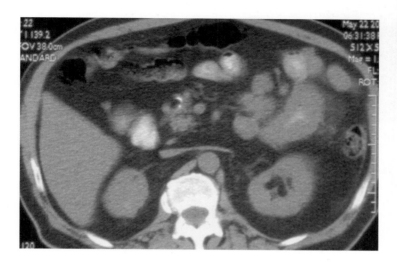

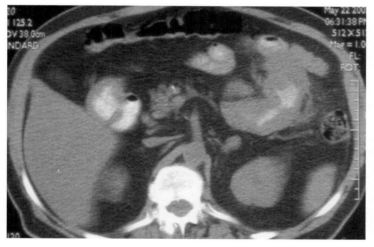

Case 46   Jejunal Adenocarcinoma

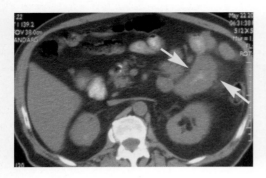 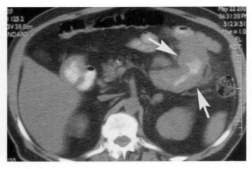

Findings

CT shows circumferential wall thickening of a short segment of proximal jejunum (arrows). The luminal margins in the affected segment are irregular. Several small lymph nodes and soft tissue stranding are seen in the adjacent mesentery.

Differential Diagnosis

▶ Lymphoma: may have a similar appearance. Aneurysmal dilation of the involved bowel segment may be present. Small bowel lymphoma is more common in the ileum than jejunum. Jejunal lymphoma may occur as a complication of celiac disease.

▶ Jejunal diverticulitis: more extensive inflammatory change with a lesser degree of wall thickening. The inflamed diverticulum is usually evident at CT and there may be associated free fluid or extraluminal air.

Teaching Points

Small bowel adenocarcinomas are uncommon. The periampullary region of the duodenum is the most common site, accounting for 55 percent of cases, followed by the jejunum (25 percent), distal duodenum (10 percent), and ileum (10 percent). Patients with small bowel adenocarcinomas have a high incidence (approximately eight times the general population) of developing a second malignancy, which is most commonly colorectal carcinoma. Small bowel adenocarcinomas occur more frequently in patients with chronic inflammatory conditions of the small bowel (celiac disease, Crohn disease, ileostomies, ileal pouches, and bypass) and inherited syndromes (familial adenomatous polyposis, hereditary nonpolyposis colon carcinoma, Peutz-Jeghers syndrome, and Neurofibromatosis type 1). On imaging, jejunal adenocarcinomas may manifest as short or long annular strictures that typically have irregular outer margins and narrow the small bowel lumen. Small lymph nodes in the adjacent small bowel mesentery are commonly present. Other imaging patterns include intraluminal polypoid masses and a focal ulcer on the mucosal surface of the small bowel.

Management

Surgical resection is the primary treatment for small bowel adenocarcinoma. Adjuvant or neoadjuvant chemotherapy may be used depending upon the tumor stage.

Further Readings

1. Buckley JA, Fishman EK. CT evaluation of small bowel neoplasms: spectrum of disease. *Radiographics*. 1998; *18*(2): 379–392.
2. Pilleul F, Penigaud M, Milot L, Saurin JC, Chayvialle JA, Valette PJ. Possible small-bowel neoplasms: contrast-enhanced and water-enhanced multidetector CT enteroclysis. *Radiology*. 2006; *241*(3): 796–801.

History

▶ 37-year-old woman with breast cancer and abdominal pain.

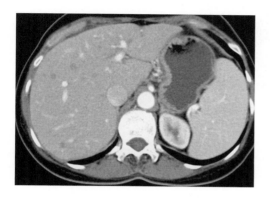

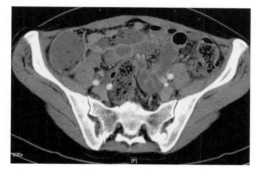

Case 47   Small Bowel Metastases

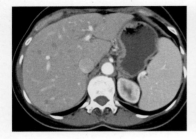 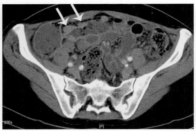 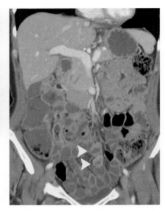

Findings

CT images (left image) show multiple hypoenhancing liver lesions consistent with metastases and (middle image) enhancing soft tissue nodules along the wall of the terminal ileum (arrows). Coronal CT image (right) shows multiple additional enhancing mural lesions (arrowheads) involving the small bowel in the mid abdomen.

Differential Diagnosis

▶ Small bowel polyps (including Peutz-Jeghers, Cronkhite-Canada syndromes): intraluminal polypoid lesions rather than mural masses.

▶ Multifocal carcinoid of the small bowel: may appear as multiple intramural or polypoid lesions. Ileal carcinoid is usually best recognized by the generally more obvious mesenteric metastasis with desmoplastic reaction, rather than the primary bowel tumor. Liver metastases from carcinoid tend to be hypervascular rather than hypovascular.

Teaching Points

Small bowel metastases account for approximately 50 percent of all small bowel neoplasms. They may arise from intraperitoneal seeding, direct extension from adjacent tumors, or hematogenous spread. The primary tumors that most commonly result in hematogenous deposition are lung cancer (particularly non-small cell), breast cancer (particularly the lobular subtype), melanoma, and renal cell carcinoma. On imaging studies, small bowel metastasis mimic the patterns of primary small bowel malignancies and may manifest short segment wall thickening, polypoid masses, or cavitary masses.

Management

Detection of small bowel metastases is difficult and requires a high index of suspicion because they are frequently asymptomatic. Endoscopy allows the potential for biopsy; however, access to the small bowel is limited. Push enteroscopy may allow more extensive access but is time-consuming and not readily available in all institutions. Treatment of small bowel metastases is typically systemic with surgery reserved for obstructing lesions.

Further Reading

1. Baker ME, Einstein DM, et al. Computed tomography enterography and magnetic resonance enterography: the future of small bowel imaging. *Clinics in Colon and Rectal Surgery*. 2008; *21*(3): 193–212.

History

▶ 57-year-old woman with longstanding abdominal cramping.

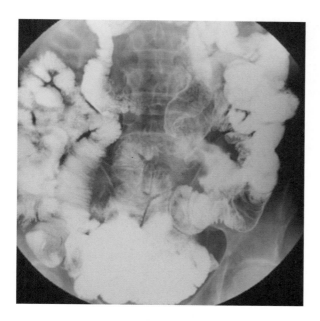

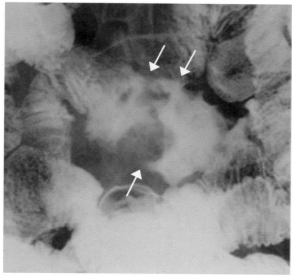

Case 48 Lymphoma in Celiac Disease (Sprue)

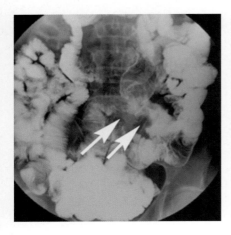 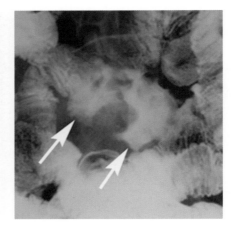

Findings

Small bowel follow through shows mild diffuse dilatation of the small bowel. There is reversal of the small bowel fold pattern with jejunization of the ileal loops in the right lower quadrant. There is aneurysmal dilatation of segment of small bowel (arrows) in the left lower quandrant that contains numerous filling defects and loss of the normal mucosal pattern

Differential Diagnosis

▶ Adenocarcinoma: more common in the proximal small intestine and may manifest as a constricting mass, filling defect, or a polypoid or ulcerated mass. Circumferential narrowing is the most common finding.

▶ GIST: intramural mass that tends to have extraluminal growth.

▶ Metastasis: may form a cavitary mass in the small bowel, but should not have the ancillary findings of sprue and the patient almost always has a known primary malignancy.

▶ Ulcerative jejunitis: rare complication of sprue that manifests as segmental wall thickening and ulceration. It may be indistinguishable from lymphoma.

Teaching Points

The distal ileum is the most common location for small bowel lymphoma because of the greater amount of lymphoid tissue in this region. Untreated or poorly controlled celiac disease, or sprue, is associated with an increased risk of associated enteropathy associated T-cell lymphoma (EATL). This subtype more frequently involves the jejunum and produces constricting lesions; however, these patients are also at increased risk for B-cell lymphomas that may affect the distal small bowel. EATL can manifest as abnormal bowel wall thickening, narrowing of the lumen, mural nodules, or an intraluminal mass. Aneurysmal dilatation is more commonly associated with B-cell lymphomas. Lymphadenopathy may be prominent, and the presence of lymphadenopathy in patients with celiac disease should suggest the possibility of complicating lymphoma.

Management

Celiac disease responds to a gluten-free diet. EATL may be treated with anthracycline-based chemotherapy agents, with or without surgery. Newer regimens including high-dose chemotherapy with autologous stem cell transplantation have achieved promising results as part of clinical trials.

Further Reading

1. Buckley O, Brien JO, et al. The imaging of celiac disease and its complications. *European Journal of Radiology*. 2008; 65(3): 483–490.

History

► 77-year-old man patient with acute abdominal pain and distention.

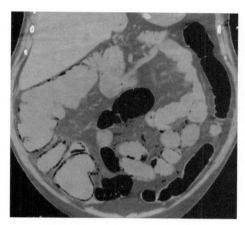

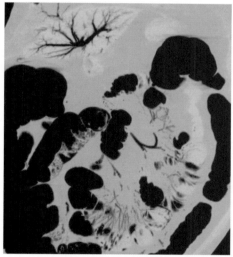

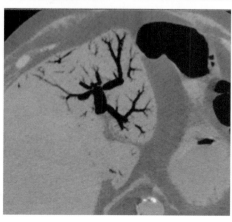

Case 49　Acute Mesenteric Ischemia

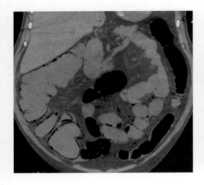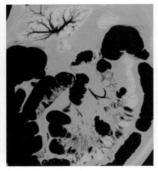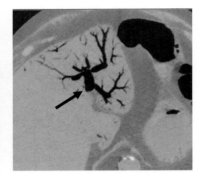

Findings

Coronal (left), coronal oblique MinIP (center) and axial MinIP (right) CT images show fluid-filled small and large bowel associated with extensive pneumatosis and portal venous and mesenteric venous gas (arrow).

Differential Diagnosis

▶ "Shock Bowel": ischemia and reperfusion of the small bowel, commonly associated with mucosal hyperenhancement, submucosal edema, and mesenteric fat stranding secondary to hypotension; usually following trauma.

▶ Benign causes of portomesenteric gas and pneumatosis: include iatrogenic (gastrostomy, sclerotherapy for gastric varices, ERCP, colonoscopy, barium enema) or a range of etiologies including collagen vascular disease, pulmonary disease, organ transplantation, seizures, steroid or cathartic therapy. Patients do not exhibit symptoms of sepsis nor acute abdomen.

Teaching Points

Acute mesenteric ischemia is caused by mesenteric arterial or venous narrowing and/or occlusion, causing inadequate perfusion. The majority of cases are related to arterial occlusion (60 to 70 percent), with embolic (atrial fibrillation, endocarditis) and atherosclerotic events being the most common cause. Suggestive CT findings include clot within the superior mesenteric artery, the superior mesenteric vein or mesenteric vessels, diminished or absent mural enhancement, and segmental mesenteric fat stranding and fluid. Bowel wall thickening may or may not be present. Venous thrombosis may be associated with diffuse mesenteric fat stranding and increased (hemorrhage or hyperemia) or decreased (edema) submucosal attenuation. Pneumatosis intestinalis is an uncommon, late and commonly irreversible finding in ischemia, suggestive of infarction.

Management

MDCT is the key imaging modality for the diagnosis of acute mesenteric ischemia, and when the disease is detected, immediate surgical consultation is indicated. In cases of primary (benign) pneumatosis or portomesenteric gas, no treatment is necessary, and spontaneous resolution often occurs within days to weeks.

Further Readings

1. Wiesner W, Mortelé KJ, Glickman JN, et al. Pneumatosis Intestinalis and Portomesenteric Venous Gas in Intestinal Ischemia: Correlation of CT Findings with Severity of Ischemia and Clinical Outcome. *Am J Roentgenol.* 2001; *177*: 1319–1323.
2. Chou CK, Mak CW, Tzeng WS, et al. CT of small bowel ischemia. *Abdom Imaging.* 2004; *29*: 18–22.

History

► 60-year-old man with right lower quadrant pain evaluated for appendicitis.

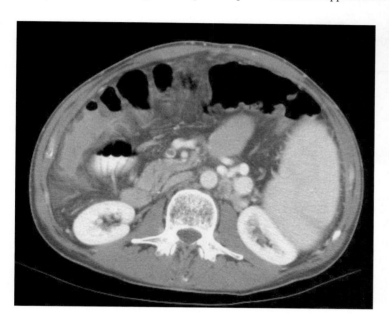

Case 50 SMV Thrombosis with Ischemic Colitis

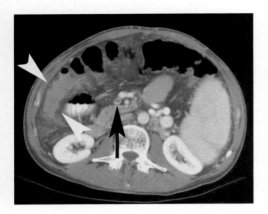

Findings

Contrast-enhanced CT shows a filling defect in a colic branch of the superior mesenteric vein (arrow). Associated ascending colon wall thickening (arrowhead) and surrounding pericolonic fat stranding suggests bowel ischemia.

Differential Diagnosis

► Pseudothrombus from early non-opacified veins: Some branches of the superior mesenteric vein opacify later than others due to different lengths of the vascular arcades. Seeing contrast fill-in on more delayed scans and lack of associated findings indicating ischemia are helpful.

Teaching Points

The causes of mesenteric ischemia and ischemic colitis can be divided into arterial and venous causes and low-flow states. Mesenteric venous thrombosis is a relatively uncommon cause of intestinal ischemia, accounting for only 15 to 20 percent of cases. The causes of mesenteric venous thrombosis include hypercoagulable states, pancreatitis, portal hypertension, cirrhosis and oral contraceptive use. In this case, the patient had a long-standing history of cirrhosis. The nonspecific clinical signs of intestinal ischemia often lead to a delay in diagnosis with significant morbidity and mortality. Traditionally, conventional angiography has been the gold standard for diagnosis. Contrast-enhanced CT currently is the diagnostic study of choice at many institutions with reported sensitivity of at least 90 percent. If a mesenteric thrombus is seen, it is important to also assess for the presence or absence of diminished bowel wall enhancement, free fluid, free intraperitoneal air, bowel wall perforation, or portal venous gas, any of which may suggest intestinal ischemia or infarction.

Management

Management of acute superior mesenteric vein thrombosis depends on the clinical as well as the radiologic findings. Surgical bowel resection may be required, but thrombectomy or transcatheter delivery of thrombolytic agents has been shown to be effective in cases without frank bowel infarction.

Further Readings

1. Bradbury MS, Kavanagh PV, Bechtold RE, et al. Mesenteric venous thrombosis: diagnosis and non-invasive imaging. *RadioGraphics.* 2002; *22*: 527–541.
2. Jancelewicz T, Vu LT, Shawo AE, Yeh B, Gasper WJ, Harris HW. Predicting strangulated small bowel obstruction: an old problem revisited. *J Gastrointest Surg.* 2009; *13*(1): 93–99.

History

▶ 17-year-old man with pelvic pain and fever.

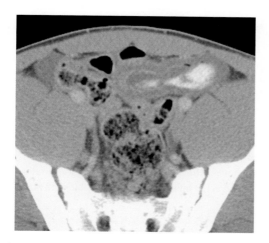

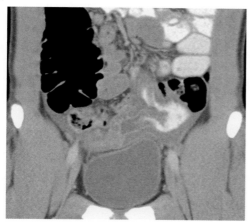

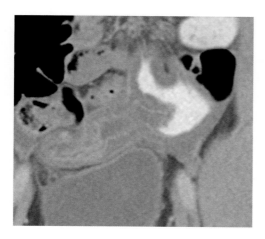

Case 51 Meckel Diverticulitis

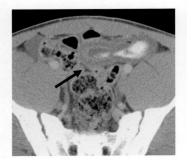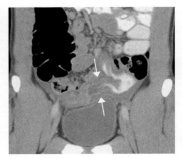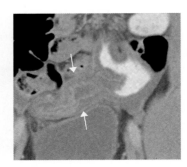

Findings

Axial (left) and coronal (center, and right in detail) contrast-enhanced CT images show a contrast-filled blind-ending diverticulum (arrow) arising from the distal small bowel. The Meckel diverticulum has mural thickening, mucosal hyperenhancement, submucosal edema and adjacent fat stranding, compatible with acute inflammation. The appendix (not shown) was normal.

Differential Diagnosis

▶ Appendicitis: distended appendix with mural thickening and hyperenhancement, occasionally with an appendicolith. It is critical to demonstrate the appendiceal origin is from the cecum and not the distal ileum.

▶ Crohn disease: diffuse thickening of the terminal ileum, with submucosal edema and mucosal hyperenhancement, associated with adjacent stranding, fistulas and/or abscesses. The appendix is seen separately, and may be secondarily involved.

Teaching Points

Meckel diverticulum is seen in approximately 2 percent of the population. It is an ileal outpouching from the embryological persistence of the omphalomesenteric (vitelline) duct. It is usually located within two feet from the ileocecal valve, measuring an average of two inches in length. Complications include diverticulitis (20 percent), bleeding, enterolith formation, inversion with or without intussusception, and obstruction (40 percent). Pathology often shows that it contains ectopic gastric or pancreatic mucosa. Secretions from the ectopic mucosa may cause peptic strictures in the distal small bowel.

Management

It is important to rule out other inflammatory causes of pelvic pain. If diagnosis is uncertain in a patient with GI bleeding, a technetium-pertechnetate scan may show accumulation of isotope in the right lower quadrant due to the presence of ectopic gastric mucosa within the diverticulum, with sensitivity more than 85 percent and specificity more than 95 percent. Pertechnetate scans are performed in children more commonly than adults because sensitivity is much lower in adults who have a broader differential diagnosis for gastrointestinal bleeding.

Further Readings

1. Elsayes DM, Menias CO, Harvin HJ, et al. Imaging Manifestations of Meckel's Diverticulum. *Am J Roentgenol.* 2007; *189*: 81–88.
2. Lee NK, Kim S, Jeon TY, et al. Complications of Congenital and Developmental Abnormalities of the Gastrointestinal Tract in Adolescents and Adults: Evaluation with Multimodality Imaging. *Radiographics.* 2010; *30*: 1489–1507.

History

▶ 54-year-old man with abdominal pain post gastric bypass surgery.

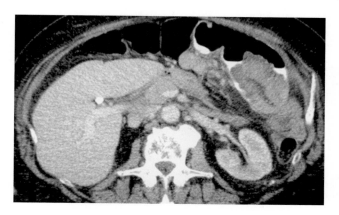

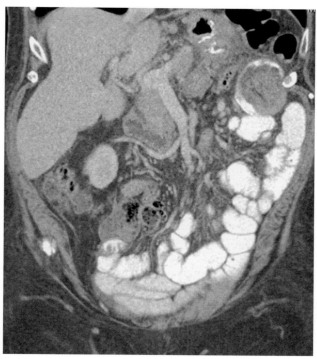

Case 52 Small Bowel Intussusception

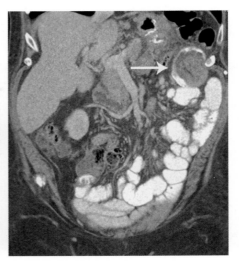

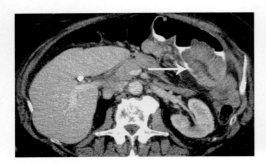

Findings

CT images show an intraluminal mass (arrow) in the proximal jejunum in the left upper quadrant. This mass contains low attenuation consistent with mesenteric fat as well as more intermediate attenuation tissue, which reflects the thickened mucosa. There is no proximal small bowel dilatation. Suture material is identified around the proximal stomach.

Differential Diagnosis

► Small bowel tumor: unlikely given the large mass, presence of fat, and the lack of small bowel obstruction.

Teaching Points

Intussusception is defined as telescoping of one part of the luminal gastrointestinal tract into an adjacent one. Symptomatic small bowel intussusception occurs most commonly in children (94 percent) where it is frequently idiopathic without an underlying cause. In symptomatic adults, an underlying cause is much more frequently encountered (80 percent) including small bowel tumors, post-operative changes (as in this case), inverted Meckel diverticulum, ectopic pancreatic tissue, or a foreign body. Small bowel intussusception may result in small bowel obstruction; however, with the advent of multidetector CT and rapid acquisition MRI sequences, transient intussusception is being identified at an increasing rate in asymptomatic individuals. Transient intussusception is typically short-segmented and does not cause proximal obstruction. On CT, intussusception has a target appearance that progresses to a sausage-shaped intraluminal mass. Eventually, a reniform mass develops due to edema of the intussusceptum. In many cases the lead point may be impossible to identify.

Management

Management depends on the clinical condition of the patient. Small bowel obstruction may respond to supportive measures. However, some patients require urgent surgery to decompress the bowel. Persistent symptomatic intussusception in adults is nearly always treated surgically, largely because of the high incidence of an underlying mass.

Further Readings

1. Byrne AT, Geoghegan T, et al. The imaging of intussusception. *Clinical Radiology.* 2005; *60*(1): 39–46.
2. Huang BY and Warshauer DM. Adult intussusception: diagnosis and clinical relevance. *Radiologic Clinics of North America*, 2003; *41*(6): 1137–1151.

History

▶ 67-year-old man with nausea, vomiting, and abdominal pain.

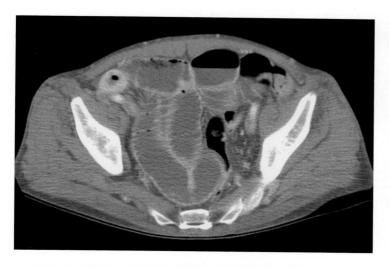

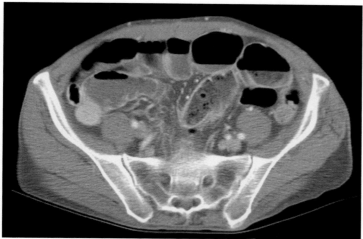

Case 53 Small Bowel Obstruction with "Small Bowel Feces Sign"

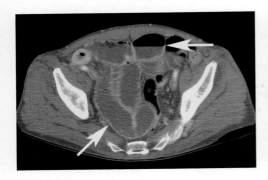 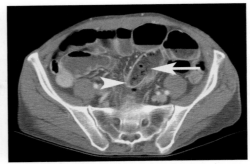

Findings

CT (left image) shows dilated fluid-filled small bowel segments (arrows) and decompressed colon. CT image of the pelvis (right image) shows intraluminal particulate material and gas within the small bowel (arrow) just proximal to the point of transition (arrowhead).

Differential Diagnosis

► Adynamic or paralytic ileus: dilated bowel without an obvious transition point to non-dilated bowel. The intraluminal content in an ileus is typically fluid or gas rather than particulate material.

► Aerophagia: dilated stomach and small bowel due to excessive swallowing of air.

Teaching Points

Small bowel obstruction accounts for approximately 4 percent of patients presenting to the emergency department with an acute abdomen. CT is currently the diagnostic test of choice for imaging suspected small bowel obstruction, with a sensitivity and specificity approaching 95 percent. The most common causes include adhesions (60 percent), hernia (15 percent), and tumor (15 percent). CT findings supporting the diagnosis of mechanical small bowel obstruction include bowel dilation greater than 3 cm and a transition point to decompressed distal small bowel. The presence of particulate material within a dilated segment of small bowel that gives the appearance of feces is termed the "small bowel feces sign." It is commonly seen just proximal to the transition point and is associated with high-grade obstruction. The proposed etiology of the small bowel feces sign is intraluminal stasis that allows for greater absorption of fluid across the bowel wall with retention of undigested food particles. It may also be seen in up to 6 percent of patients without bowel obstruction.

Management

Low-grade or partial small bowel obstructions can be managed conservatively with nasogastric suction, intravenous fluids, and bowel rest. CT findings of a closed loop obstruction, free intraperitoneal air, bowel wall pneumatosis, delayed bowel wall enhancement, or portal venous gas necessitate immediate surgery for resection of ischemic or necrotic bowel.

Further Reading

1. Mayo-Smith WW, Wittenberg J, Bennett GL, Gervais DA, Gazelle GS, Mueller PR. The CT small bowel faeces sign: description and clinical significance. *Clin Radiol.* 1995; *50*: 765–767.

History

▸ 70-year-old woman with abdominal pain.

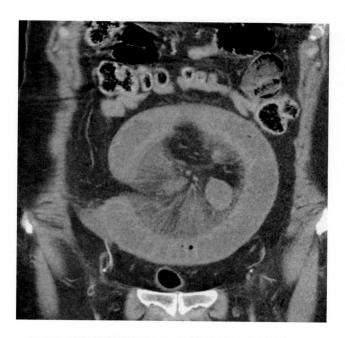

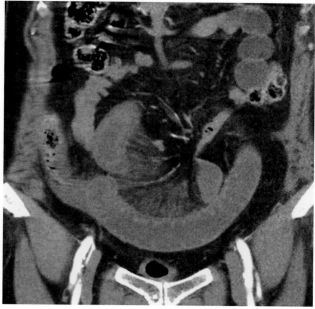

Case 54 Closed-Loop Small Bowel Obstruction

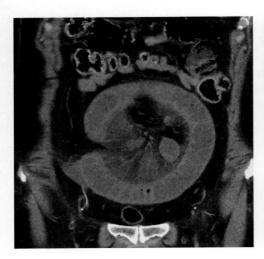 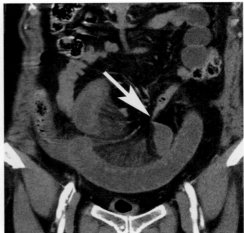

Findings

Coronal CT images show a C-shaped dilated segment of small bowel in the central abdomen, with two adjacent transition points at the mesenteric root on either end of the dilated bowel, and distal decompressed bowel (arrow). Hypoenhancement and wall thickening of the dilated small bowel segment as well as mesenteric fat stranding and adjacent free fluid are all suggestive of ischemia due to strangulation.

Differential Diagnosis

▶ Small bowel ileus: results in dilated loops of small bowel but without a transition point. Often diffuse and involves the large bowel as well as the small bowel.

▶ Simple small bowel obstruction: may resemble a closed loop obstruction, but only one transition point should be found.

Teaching Points

Although some small bowel obstructions may be managed conservatively, particularly when they are simple and do not appear high-grade or complete, closed-loop obstructions are considered a surgical emergency due to a higher risk of ischemia, surgical complications, morbidity, and hospital stay duration. Closed-loop obstruction may be due to small bowel volvulus where both bowel and its mesenteric vessels can be seen to twist upon themselves by more than 180 degrees ("whirlpool sign"). In this case, multiple bowel transition points may be seen close to each other in the mesenteric root. Small bowel herniation or adhesions may also cause closed loop obstructions. Signs of mesenteric ischemia include segmental mesenteric root edema, free fluid, mural nonenhancement, and pneumatosis intestinalis.

Management

Closed-loop small bowel obstruction is a surgical emergency, especially when there are clinical or radiological signs of intestinal ischemia.

Further Readings

1. Sandhu PS, Joe BN, Coakley FV, Qayyum A, Webb EM, Yeh BM. Bowel transition points: multiplicity and posterior location at CT are associated with small-bowel volvulus. *Radiology*. 2007; *245*(1): 160–167.
2. Qalbani A, Paushter D, Dachman AH. Multidetector row CT of small bowel obstruction. *Radiologic Clinics of North America*. 2007; *45*: 499–512.

History

▶ 58-year-old woman complains of bloating, abdominal distension, diarrhea, and abdominal pain.

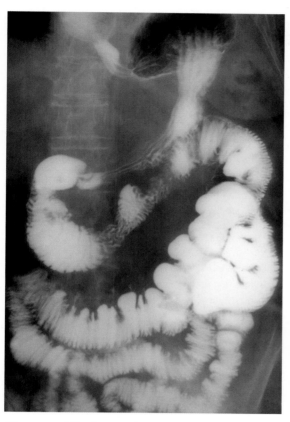

(Courtesy of Charles A. Rohrmann, Jr., MD, Seattle, WA)

Case 55 Scleroderma

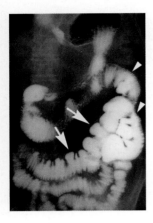

Findings

Small bowel follow through image shows proximal small bowel distension, increased number and crowding of the folds (arrowheads), and wide-mouthed sacculations (arrows) along the mesenteric border. At the superior edge of the image, there is gastroesophageal reflux and dilatation of the distal esophagus.

Differential Diagnosis

▶ Jejunal diverticulosis: characterized by acquired sacculations along the mesenteric border. The sacculations may be numerous and accompanied by bowel distension and dysmotility. The unaffected portion of the small bowel may appear normal.

▶ Crohn disease: sacculations are present in advanced disease and are associated with fibrotic straightening and shortening of the mesenteric border with redundancy and sacculations of the antimesenteric border. Other features of Crohn disease are usually apparent.

▶ Prior surgery: sacculations and luminal dilatation may occur at or near surgical anastomosis.

Teaching Points

Patients with collagen vascular disorders (scleroderma, mixed connective tissue disease, dermatomyositis, polymyositis, and systemic lupus erythematosis) develop malabsorption and dysmotility from small bowel involvement. Scleroderma has the most characteristic and impressive radiologic features throughout the gastrointestinal tract. Clinically, patients may experience vomiting and abdominal distension that may mimic mechanical obstruction. The small bowel is classically dilated with a crowded, pronounced fold pattern that has been called the "hidebound bowel" sign. The pattern of crowded folds is related to collagen deposition in the circular muscle layer of the muscularis propria. Duodenal dilatation may be a prominent feature. Focal areas of muscular thinning with collagen deposition and fibrosis are responsible for the sacculations that frequently occur in the small and large bowel.

Management

Nutritional support and prokinetics are used to manage intestinal symptoms. For patients who do not respond, octreotide or parenteral nutrition may be necessary.

Further Readings

1. Rohrmann CA, Jr., Ricci MT, Krishnamurthy S, Schuffler MD. Radiologic and histologic differentiation of neuromuscular disorders of the gastrointestinal tract: visceral myopathies, visceral neuropathies, and progressive systemic sclerosis. *Am J Roentgenol.* 1984; *143*(5): 933–941.
2. Pickhardt PJ. The "hide-bound" bowel sign. *Radiology.* 1999; *213*(3): 837–838.

History

▶ 57-year-old man with abdominal pain and fever.

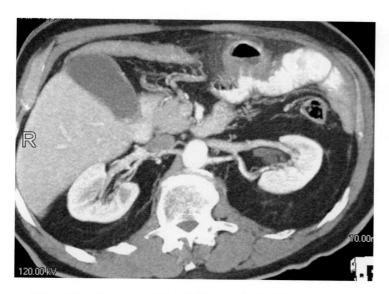

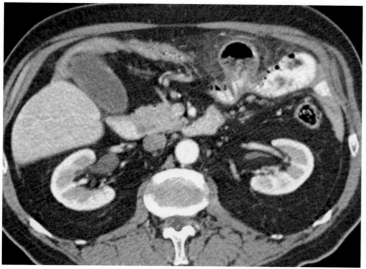

Case 56   Jejunal Diverticulitis

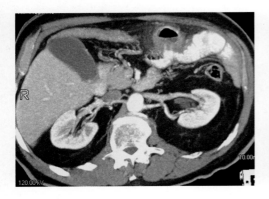 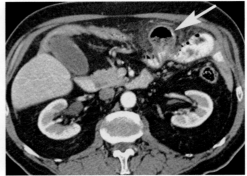

Findings

CT shows a diverticular outpouching (arrow) that communicates with the proximal jejunum. It has a mildly thickened wall and contains debris. There is inflammatory stranding surrounding the diverticulum. No extraluminal gas.

Differential Diagnosis

► Cavitary neoplasm: exoenteric growth of small bowel tumors such as gastrointestinal stromal tumor, lymphoma, metastatic disease, and rarely, adenocarcinoma may have a similar appearance. Tumors typically have a thicker and more irregular wall and lack surrounding inflammatory change.
► Crohn disease with sacculations: sacculations in Crohn disease occur on the antimesenteric border because of straightening and shortening of the mesenteric border from chronic inflammation. Other features of Crohn disease are usually present.
► Meckel diverticulitis: diagnosed by location in the distal ileum.

Teaching Points

Jejunal and ileal diverticula are acquired protrusions of mucosa and submucosa along the mesenteric border. In contrast, Meckel diverticulum is located on the anti-mesenteric border of the distal ileum and is composed of all layers of the bowel wall. Acquired diverticula may occur in the jejunum and ileum. Although most are idiopathic, they may occur in association with motility disorders that affect the smooth muscle or myenteric plexus in the bowel wall. Acquired small bowel diverticula are generally round, variable in size, and have a wide mouth. The majority of patients are asymptomatic. Bacterial overgrowth with resultant malabsorption may occur when there is extensive small bowel diverticulosis. Other complications include diverticulitis with or without perforation, obstruction, and gastrointestinal bleeding. Uncomplicated small bowel diverticula are thin-walled outpouchings. Intraluminal small bowel contents or contrast fill the diverticular lumen. Inflamed diverticula tend to have thicker wall with inflammatory changes and/or fluid in the adjacent mesentery. Oral contrast may not enter the diverticular lumen in diverticulitis because of obstruction at the neck of the diverticulum. Occasionally the inflamed diverticulum may appear mass-like. The presence of extraluminal gas indicates perforation.

Management

Similar to appendicitis and Meckel diverticulitis, small bowel diverticulitis is managed with surgical resection.

Further Reading

1. Coulier B, Maldague P, Bourgeois A, Broze B. Diverticulitis of the small bowel: CT diagnosis. *Abdom Imaging.* 2007; *32*(2): 228–233.

Part 5 — Appendix

History

▶ 54-year-old man was initially evaluated for an incidentally discovered right lower quadrant mass on ultrasound. He now presents approximately one year later with abdominal distention.

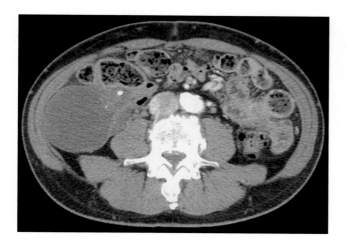

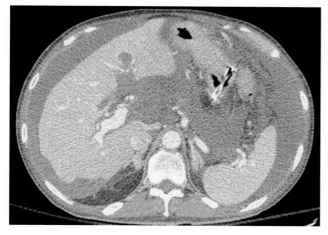

Case 57 Mucinous Adenocarcinoma of the Appendix with Pseudomyxoma Peritonei

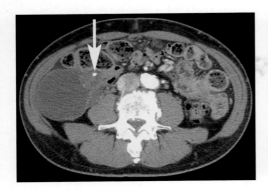 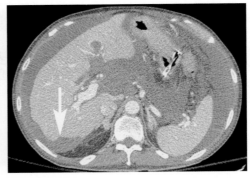

Findings

CT (left) shows a mixed solid and cystic mass abutting and displacing the cecum with irregular mural thickening and calcification (white arrow). A normal appendix was not visualized. Subsequent CT (right) shows pseudomyxoma peritonei as shown by intraperitoneal fluid-attenuation masses "scalloping" the liver margin (white arrow) and other organs.

Differential Diagnosis

- ▸ Peritoneal carcinomatosis: characterized by omental caking and soft tissue nodularity along serosal surfaces.
- ▸ Bacterial peritonitis: complex ascites with peritoneal enhancement and intra-abdominal fat stranding with symptoms of sepsis.

Teaching Points

Mucoceles of the appendix may be due to non-neoplastic chronic inflammatory obstruction of the appendix (simple mucocele or retention cyst) or from mucin-producing neoplasms (appendiceal mucinous cystadenoma or cystadenocarcinoma). Marked appendiceal distention is common in mucin-producing tumors. On CT, a mucin-producing tumor of the appendix produces cystic dilatation of the appendix with or without mural nodularity. Curvilinear mural calcification is common in cystadenomas. Mural nodularity raises suspicion of cystadenocarcinoma. Pseudomyxoma peritonei is produced by low-grade mucinous cystadenocarciomas of the appendix. It is characterized by the accumulation of intraperitoneal mucinous material on the omental and peritoneal surfaces.

Management

Non-ruptured appendiceal mucoceles are typically treated with surgical resection. Benign mucoceles and cystadenomas carry a good prognosis, while cystadenocarcinomas typically have a poorer outcome. Pseudomyxoma peritonei is difficult to treat, but symptoms of mass effect can be mitigated by surgical debulking with or without adjuvant intraperitoneal chemotherapy.

Further Reading

1. Pickhardt PJ, Levy AD, Rohrmann CA Jr, and Kende AI. Primary Neoplasms of the Appendix: Radiologic Spectrum of Disease with Pathologic Correlation. *RadioGraphics*. 2003; 23: 645–662.

History

▶ 66-year-old man with right lower quadrant pain.

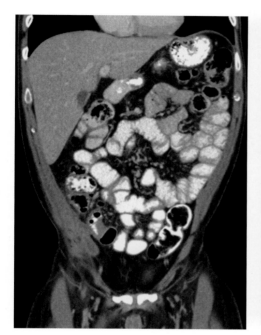 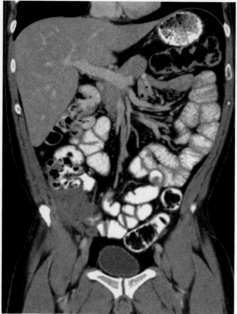

Case 58 Appendiceal Lymphoma

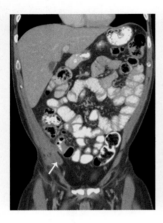
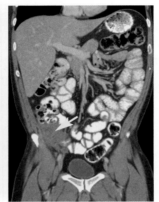

Findings

CT shows a homogeneous attenuation soft tissue mass (arrow) in the region of the proximal appendix that extends to involve the base of the cecum. The distal appendix is dilated.

Differential Diagnosis

▶ Appendicitis: appendiceal dilatation with mural thickening suggests the diagnosis of appendicitis, but the presence of a large soft tissue mass is not a feature of primary inflammatory appendicitis.

▶ Appendiceal adenocarcinoma: may have an identical appearance. Tends to be more heterogeneous in CT attenuation than lymphoma.

Teaching Points

Although the gastrointestinal tract is the most common extranodal site for non-Hodgkin's lymphoma, the appendix is not commonly a site of disease. The appendix may be a primary or secondary site for lymphoma. The majority of patients present to clinical attention with signs and symptoms similar to acute appendicitis. The CT findings of appendiceal lymphoma are similar to lymphoma elsewhere in the gastrointestinal tract: diffuse enlargement of the appendix with homogeneous attenuation mural thickening, polypoid or infiltrating mass, or aneurysmal dilatation of the appendiceal lumen in a thick-walled appendix. If the lymphoma obstructs the appendiceal lumen, secondary changes of appendicitis may also be present. Soft tissue infiltration in the periappendical fat may represent lymphomatous infiltration or inflammatory stranding from appendiceal obstruction. Similar CT findings may also be seen in other appendiceal primary tumors such as adenocarcinoma and neuroendocrine neoplasms. The finding of aneurysmal dilatation of a thickened appendix and the ancillary finding of bulky abdominal or retroperitoneal lymphadenopathy adds specificity to the diagnosis.

Management

Non-Hodgkin gastrointestinal lymphomas are primarily managed with various chemotherapeutic regimens that are dependent upon the specific lymphoma subtype. Surgical intervention may occur to manage complications such as bowel obstruction.

Further Reading

1. Pickhardt PJ, Levy AD, Rohrmann CA, Jr., Abbondanzo SL, Kende AI. Non-Hodgkin's lymphoma of the appendix: clinical and CT findings with pathologic correlation. *Am J Roentgenol.* 2002 May;*178*(5):1123–1127.

History

▶ 28-year-old man with right inguinal and scrotal pain and tenderness.

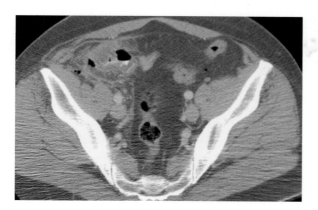

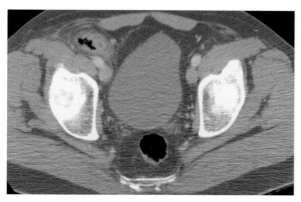

Case 59 Amyand's Syndrome: Acute Appendicitis in an Inguinal Hernia

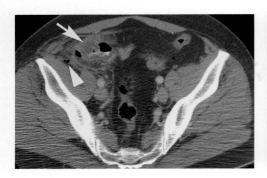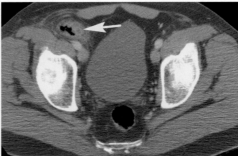

Findings

CT images show a right inguinal hernia containing the cecum (arrow on left image), which has a low attenuation thickened wall with surrounding inflammatory stranding. Medial to the cecum, in the inguinal canal, is a small rim-enhancing structure (arrow on right image) that represents the inflamed appendix.

Differential Diagnosis

▶ Incarcerated or strangulated inguinal hernia: may have an identical appearance. The distinction can only be made if the inflamed appendix is visualized.

Teaching Points

Named after Claudius Amyand, the surgeon of King George II who performed the first successful recorded appendectomy in 1735, Amyand's hernia is an inguinal hernia containing the appendix. The appendix may be normal, inflamed, perforated, or harbor a neoplasm. More common in adult men, the hernia has also been reported in the pediatric population. The clinical presentation of appendicitis in Amyand's hernia (Amyand's Syndrome) is usually indistinguishable from an incarcerated hernia. Preoperative imaging with CT may establish the diagnosis when an inflamed appendix is identified within the hernia sac.

Management

The surgical management for Amyand's hernia varies based upon whether the appendix is normal or inflamed. If the appendix is normal, reduction and repair of the hernia with or without appendectomy may be performed. Prosthetic materials may be used if indicated. In the case of appendicitis, appendectomy, reduction of the hernia, and repair of the hernia without prosthetic material are often performed.

Further Readings

1. Milanchi S, Allins AD. Amyand's hernia: history, imaging, and management. *Hernia*. 2008 Jun;*12*(3):321–322.
2. Luchs JS, Halpern D, Katz DS. Amyand's hernia: prospective CT diagnosis. *J Comput Assist Tomogr*. 2000; *24*(6):884–886.

History

▶ 21-year-old man with 72-hour history of abdominal pain, fever and leukocytosis.

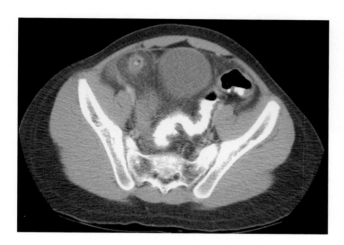

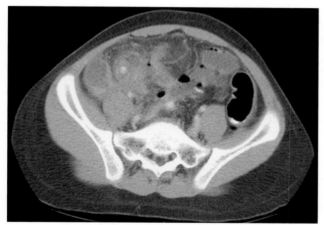

Case 60   Acute Appendicitis

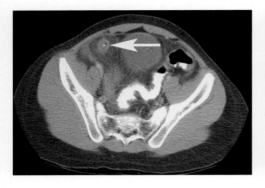 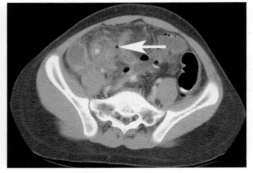

Findings

CT (left) shows a dilated thick-walled tubular structure in the right lower quadrant with mural hyperenhancement (arrow), associated free fluid, fat stranding and an intraluminal calcification (appendicolith). Slightly more cephalad CT (right) shows an extraluminal focus of gas (arrow).

Differential Diagnosis

▶ Meckel's diverticulitis: blind-ending tubular structure that usually arises from the ileum, often has gastric mucosa, and is prone to bleeding.
▶ Mesenteric adenitis: right lower quadrant lymphadenopathy with or without associated ileal wall thickening.
▶ Active Crohn disease: ileal inflammation, often with skip lesions or fistulas.

Teaching Points

Acute appendicitis is common and requires surgical consultation to minimize morbidity. While appendicitis can occur at any age, the peak incidence is in young adulthood. The ACR Appropriateness Criteria for suspected appendicitis recommend contrast-enhanced CT in most cases, but right lower quadrant ultrasound with graded compression is considered the initial study of choice in pregnant patients and in children less than 14 years of age. Use of oral or rectal contrast to aid in the diagnosis is based on institutional preference, without clear consensus. Key CT findings include the finding of a dilated (greater than 6 mm), enhancing, blind-ending tubular structure arising from the cecum with associated mesoappendiceal fat stranding and sometimes presence of an appendicolith. Appendiceal rupture should be suspected in the presence of surrounding inflammatory fluid collections, extraluminal gas or associated small bowel obstruction.

Management

Most cases of acute appendicitis are managed with laparoscopic or open appendectomy. Nonsurgical management with antibiotics has shown anecdotal success, but recurrence is a concern. Increasingly, patients with associated peri-appendiceal abscess are being managed temporarily with percutaneous drainage.

Further Reading

1. van Randen A, Bipat S, Zwinderman AH, Ubbink DT, Stoker J, Boermeester MA. Acute appendicitis: meta-analysis of diagnostic performance of CT and graded compression US related to prevalence of disease. *Radiology.* 2008; *249*(1):97–106.

Part 6   Colon, Rectum, and Anus

History

▶ 61-year-old man with left lower quadrant pain and fever. Initial CT scan (top), and follow-up scan two months later (bottom).

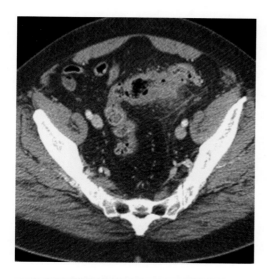

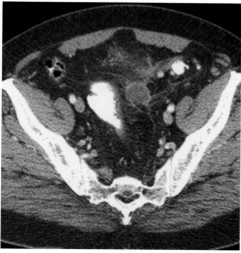

Case 61 Complicated Diverticulitis

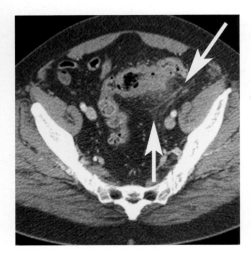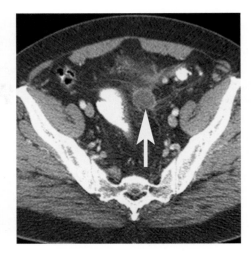

Findings

Initial CT (left) shows focally thickened and hyperenhancing sigmoid wall with multiple diverticula and surrounding inflammatory stranding (arrows) in the sigmoid mesocolon. The follow-up CT (right) with rectal contrast shows a new rim-enhancing abscess (arrow) in the sigmoid mesocolon.

Differential Diagnosis

▶ Colon carcinoma: presence of lymphadenopathy, focal mass, or minimal inflammatory changes.
▶ Epiploic appendagitis: less than 3 cm fatty mass with rim sign and central engorged vessel.
▶ Ischemic colitis: Typically segmental distribution with poor bowel wall enhancement.

Teaching Points

Colonic diverticulosis is common in Western society due to low fiber diets. It typically affects patients older than 50 years. Colonic diverticula are small (0.5 to 1cm) outpouchings of the colonic mucosa and submucosa through the muscular layer and most common in the sigmoid colon, but they can occur throughout the colon. Acute diverticulitis is caused by an obstructed diverticulum with subsequent inflammation. The diagnosis is made by the CT findings of colonic wall thickening and hyperemia with inflammatory changes in the pericolonic fat. The inflamed diverticula may be visualized. Perforation and abscess formation occur in up to 30 percent of cases. Other complications of diverticulitis include colonic obstruction, fistulas to bladder or other organs, and peritonitis. Rarely, one can see liver or pulmonary abscesses from hematogenous bacterial spread, and gas or thrombus may be found in mesenteric and portal veins. While unusual, an underlying colon cancer is difficult to exclude.

Management

In acute diverticulitis, antibiotics are given and percutaneous CT-guided abscess drainage or surgery may be required if perforation is seen. Follow-up endoscopic visualization is commonly recommended after the acute stage to exclude an underlying malignancy.

Further Readings

1. Hortan KM, Corl FM, Fishman EK. CT evaluation of the colon: inflammatory disease. *RadioGraphics* 2000; *20*(2):399–418.
2. Zaidi E, Daly B. CT and Clinical features of acute diverticulitis in an urban U.S. Population: rising frequency in young, obese adults. *Am J Roentgenol.* 2006; *17*: 689–694.

History

▸ 31-year-old woman presenting with severe left lower quadrant pain and fever.

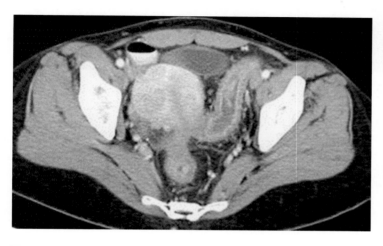

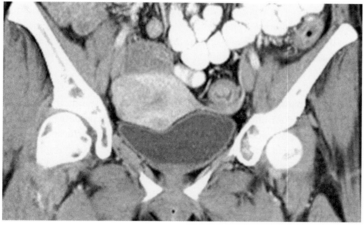

Case 62 Ulcerative Colitis with Inflammatory Pseudopolyps

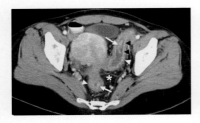 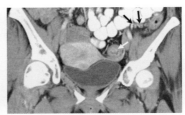 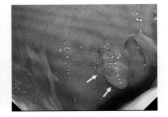

Findings

CT images obtained during the portal venous phase show two enhancing mucosal lesions in the rectum and sigmoid colon (white arrows). Mucosal hyperenhancement (black arrowheads) and mural stratification are present along with circumferential and symmetric bowel wall thickening (white arrowhead), pericolonic stranding (white asterisks), and mesenteric hyperemia (black arrow). Colonoscopy images of the sigmoid colon (right) confirm the presence of the polypoid mucosal lesion (white arrows).

Differential Diagnosis

► Inflammatory polyps: in the setting of active disease, true polyps and pseudopolyps frequently coexist because the residual mucosa that forms pseudopolyps is often inflamed.
► Post-inflammatory polyps: appear during the non-active phase of disease. These polyps are often long and thin (filiform), almost always multiple, and may have an unusual clubbed, branching or bridging appearance.
► Adenocarcinoma: arises from regions of dysplasia and tends to be flat or infiltrative. Can appear as a narrowed segment with an eccentric lumen and irregular contour.

Teaching Points

Ulcerative colitis is a common idiopathic inflammatory bowel disease with concentric and symmetric colonic involvement beginning in the rectum with continuous proximal progression. It is a predominantly mucosal and submucosal disease with the active phase appearing as mural thickening and stratification with mesenteric hyperemia and mucosal hyperenhancement. Erosion into the mucosa and submucosa results in characteristic collar-button ulcers on fluoroscopic images. When more extensive ulcerations develop and coalesce, regions of mucosa slough off leaving scattered islands of relatively normal mucosa called pseudopolyps. In active ulcerative colitis, small islands of inflamed mucosa form inflammatory polyps. Post inflammatory polyps form as the extensive ulcerations heal and epithelium regenerates.

Management

Patients with ulcerative colitis are at an increased risk for adenocarcinoma. Although pseudopolyps and inflammatory polyps have no malignant potential, differentiating these polyps from adenocarcinoma and dysplasia is sometimes difficult or impossible. In these cases, endoscopy and biopsy should be recommended for definitive diagnosis of suspicious lesions.

Further Reading

1. Buck JL, Dachman AH, Sobin LH. Polypoid and pseudopolypoid manifestations of inflammatory bowel disease. *RadioGraphics* 1991; *11*: 293–304.

History

► 45-year-old woman with diarrhea.

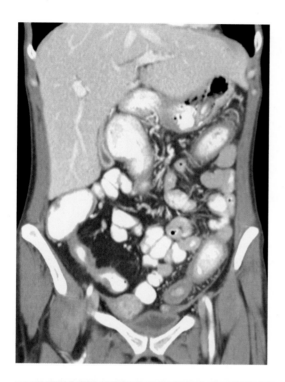

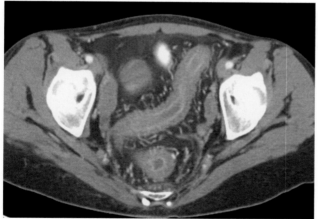

Case 63 Crohn's Colitis

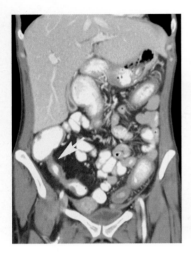
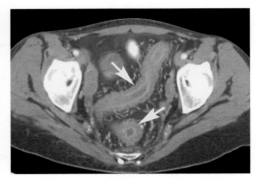

Findings

Coronal CT shows long segment narrowing of the terminal ileum with wall thickening (arrow on left image). A short stricture is also present in the distal ileum. The sigmoid colon wall is thickened. The axial CT shows mural thickening and mucosal hyperenhancement of the rectosigmoid colon (arrows on right image). There is also engorgement of the vasa recta supplying the rectosigmoid.

Differential Diagnosis

► Ulcerative colitis: may involve the rectum and sigmoid only. It should not have discontinuous involvement of the terminal ileum.
► Infectious colitis: generally does not cause narrowing or structuring of the terminal ileum. The exception is tuberculosis.
► Radiation colitis: can involve both the small bowel and colon, but patient has history of prior radiation and the involved bowel loops are located in the radiation port area.
► Graft-versus-host disease: can involve both the small bowel and colon, but patient has history of prior transplantation, especially bone marrow transplantation.

Teaching Points

The distinction between ulcerative colitis and Crohn disease involving the colon can be difficult. CT findings to suggest Crohn colitis include concomitant involvement of the small bowel and extraluminal complications such as abscess and fistula formation. Skip lesions are a distinctive feature of Crohn disease whereas continuous inflammation from the rectum proximally is typical of ulcerative colitis. The mean wall thickness is reportedly greater and more homogeneous in Crohn colitis than in ulcerative colitis. Other findings on CT to suggest Crohn disease include fibrofatty proliferation, perianal fistulizing disease, and abscess formation.

Management

The treatment includes bowel rest, steroids, antibiotics, and immunosuppression. Surgical resection of strictures may be necessary in some patients.

Further Readings

1. Joffe, N., Antonioli, D, et al. Focal Granulomatous (Crohn's) Colitis: Radiologic-Pathologic Correlation. *Abdom Imaging,* Volume 3, 1:73–80. 1978.
2. Gore, R, Marn, C, et al. CT Findings in Ulcerative, granulomatous and indeterminate colitis. *Am J Roentgenol. 143*(2): 279–284. 1984.

History

▶ 60-year-old man with diarrhea, abdominal distension, leukocytosis, and recent antibiotic treatment for necrotizing fasciitis of the leg.

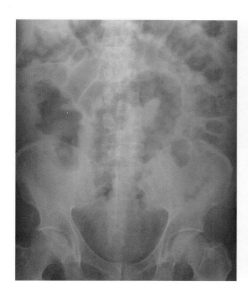
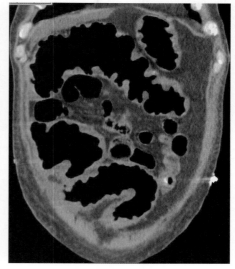
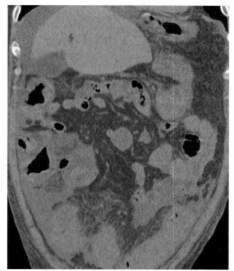

Case 64 Pseudomembranous Colitis

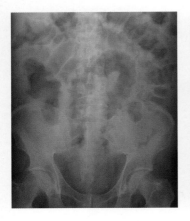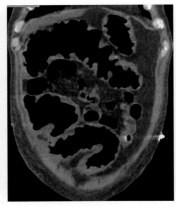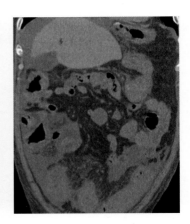

Findings

Abdominal radiograph (left) and anterior coronal noncontrast CT (middle) show dilated gas-filled colon with marked wall thickening including thumbprinting and pseudopolyp formation. A more posterior coronal CT image (right) shows free peritoneal fluid, thick-walled sigmoid colon, and pericolonic fat stranding.

Differential Diagnosis

► Ischemic colitis: most common in the elderly and may be diffuse or segmental when the watershed areas of the splenic flexure or rectosigmoid are affected.
► Infectious colitis: may be radiographically indistinguishable from other colitides and requires stool sampling for diagnosis.
► Inflammatory bowel disease: Crohn disease and ulcerative colitis tend to have less wall thickening, pericolonic inflammation, and ascites.

Teaching Points

Pseudomembranous colitis should be suspected in any patient with diarrhea or other abdominal symptoms who has been undergoing antibiotic treatment within recent months. Broad-spectrum antibiotics allow *Clostricum difficile* to proliferate and elaborate a toxin that causes the colitis. CT and abdominal radiographic findings include diffuse colonic wall thickening, which may include thumbprinting and a polypoid-like appearance of the haustral folds. Toxic megacolon and perforation may occur. In advanced stages, ascites and pericolonic fat stranding is present on CT. Low attenuation mural thickening corresponding to mucosal and submucosal edema can appear as a "target" when the bowel is seen in cross-section on intravenous contras-enhanced images, and may give the appearance of an "accordion" when viewed longitudinal to the bowel. These findings, however, are not specific to pseudomembranous colitis and may be seen in other causes of colonic edema and inflammation.

Management

Surgical intervention with colectomy may be required for refractory cases or when toxic megacolon or pneumatosis complicate the disease.

Further Readings

1. Brunner D, Feifarek C, McNeely D, Haney P. CT of pseudomembranous colitis. *Gastrointest Radiol*. 1984; 9:73–75.
2. Kawamoto S, Horton KM, Fishman EK. Pseudomembranous colitis: spectrum of imaging findings with clinical and pathologic correlation. *RadioGraphics*. 1999; 19:877–897.

History

▶ 22-year-old man with leukemia who presents with bloody stool, diarrhea, and abdominal pain.

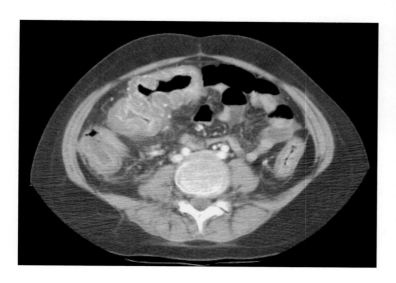

Case 65 Cytomegalovirus Colitis

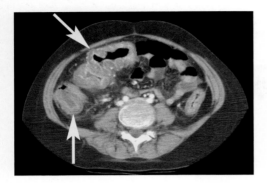

Findings

Axial contrast-enhanced CT image of the abdomen shows diffuse colonic mural thickening, particularly of the cecum and ascending colon (arrows). Pericolonic fat stranding is present.

Differential Diagnosis

- ▶ Neutropenic colitis (typhlitis): colonic wall thickening and pericolonic inflammation involving the cecum and ascending colon.
- ▶ Pseudomembranous colitis: typically involves the whole colon. Patient often has history of antibiotic use.
- ▶ Tuberculosis: may have indolent presentation and low-density mesenteric lymph nodes.
- ▶ Inflammatory bowel disease: usually shows rectal involvement without skip lesions.

Teaching Points

Between 50 and 80 percent of the world population is seropositive for cytomegalovirus (CMV). Initial infection in an immunocompetent host is typically mild and may be subclinical. Patients with impairment of immune function from acquired immunodeficiency syndrome (AIDS) or immunosuppressive therapy after organ transplant are susceptible to reactivation with viral proliferation and severe systemic illness. CMV colitis has been reported in 3 to 5 percent of AIDS patients and 2 to 16 percent of post-transplant patients. CT findings include cecal wall thickening with contiguous involvement of the terminal ileum and ascending colon. Mucosal ulcerations are frequent and may erode into adjacent blood vessels with resultant hemorrhage into the bowel wall or lumen. Persistent bowel wall inflammation can result in vascular compromise with ischemia/necrosis, potential bowel perforation, and peritonitis.

Management

Treatment with the antiviral medication gancyclovir is first-line therapy for immunocompetent and immunocompromised patients. For patients with AIDS, concurrent use of antiretrovirals has been shown to augment treatment by boosting the patient's immune response.

Further Readings

1. Frager DH, Frager JD, Wolf EL, et al. Cytomegalovirus Colitis in Acquired Immune Deficiency Syndrome: Radiologic Spectrum. *Gastrointest Radiol.* 1986;*11*(3):241–246.
2. Maconi G, Colombo E, Zerbi P, et al. Prevalence, Detection Rate and Outcome of Cytomegalovirus Infection in Ulcerative Colitis Patients Requiring Colonic Resection. *Dig Liver Dis.* 2005; *37*(6): 418–423.
3. Schmit M, Bethge W, Beck R, Faul C, Claussen CD, Horger M. CT of Gastrointestinal Complications Associated with Hematopoietic Stem Cell Transplantation. *Am J Roentgenol.* 2008; *190*: 712–719.

History

▶ 62-year-old man post bone marrow transplant presenting with abdominal pain, fever, and diarrhea.

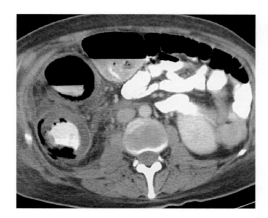
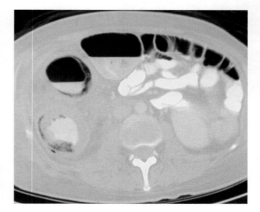
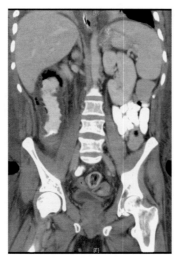

Case 66 Neutropenic Colitis (Typhlitis)

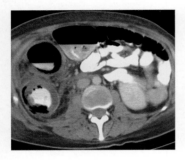 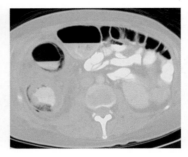 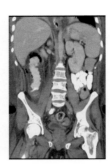

Findings

CT images show marked cecal and ascending colon wall thickening, pericolonic inflammation, and pneumatosis. The suspected pneumatosis is confirmed on lung windows (middle). Fluid is tracking in the ileocolic mesentery. There is no pneumoperitoneum, complicating obstruction, or involvement of the small bowel.

Differential Diagnosis

▶ Pseudomembranous colitis (PMC): altered gut flora following antibiotic therapy allows for *C. difficile* colonization. Marked low attenuation wall thickening, and pancolitis, commonly characterize PMC. No small bowel involvement.

▶ Graft-versus-host disease: occurs early following bone marrow transplant. Common features include extensive dilatation and mucosal hyperenhancement. Wall thickening is typically less pronounced. History of bone marrow transplant is key.

▶ Crohn disease: Features include discontinuity of disease, terminal ileal involvement, strictures, fistulas, and lymph node enlargement. Pneumatosis is rare.

▶ Infectious colitis: there is significant overlap in the imaging features including bowel wall thickening, pericolonic stranding, and ascites. Pneumatosis is rare. Certain pathogens characteristically involve the right colon with and without ileal involvement; these include *Salmonella, Yersinia, Tuberculosis,* and *Amebiasis.*

Teaching Points

Causes of neutropenia include drug reactions, autoimmune diseases, infections, and hematologic malignancies. Neutropenic colitis remains poorly understood and pathologically is represented by compromised wall integrity with subsequent bacterial or fungal invasion. Neutropenic colitis has been reported in all segments of the large bowel; however, it is most commonly located within the cecum. Suggestive CT findings include bowel wall thickening, pericolonic stranding, ascites and cecal pneumatosis. Severe cases may result in any combination of abscess formation, sepsis, intestinal necrosis, hemorrhage, and perforation.

Management

In the setting of a history of neutropenia, a prompt diagnosis is essential. Treatment with supportive therapy including broad-spectrum antibiotics and supplemental nutrition is necessary. Surgical resection may be required.

Further Reading

1. Kirkpatrick I, Greenberg H. Gastrointestinal Complications in the Neutropenic Patient: Characterization and Differentiation. *Radiology* 2003;*226*:668–674.

History

► 78-year-old man with abdominal pain and elevated lactate.

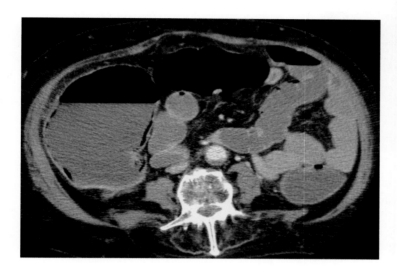

Case 67   Ischemic Colitis

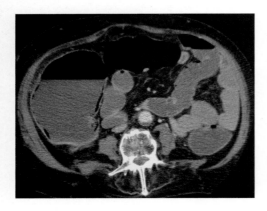

Findings

CT shows a dilated, fluid-filled cecum with submucosal pneumatosis and mild pericolonic stranding.

Differential Diagnosis

► Infectious colitis or inflammatory bowel disease: usually cause significant bowel wall thickening and a target or double halo sign from submucosal edema and mucosal hyperenhancement. Pneumatosis usually is not a characteristic feature unless toxic megacolon is present.

► Other causes of pneumatosis include: post invasive procedure such as colonoscopy, idiopathic, cystic fibrosis, scleroderma, chemotherapeutic agents, and steroid therapy.

Teaching Points

The incidence of ischemic colitis is not entirely known because the majority of cases are transient and resolve spontaneously. Ischemic colitis most often affects elderly patients and is associated with nonspecific symptoms such as vague abdominal pain, bleeding, and/or diarrhea. Serum lactate may be elevated, and the patient may also have an increased white cell count and a metabolic acidosis. Possible causes include systemic hypoperfusion, venous thrombosis, arterial occlusion, embolism, and vasculitis. Ischemic colitis tends to occur in the watershed area of the colon: splenic flexure or rectosigmoid junction. Most cases heal without sequela; however, strictures may develop in severe cases. On CT, the ability to diagnose ischemia from other causes of bowel wall thickening may be difficult. A high index of suspicion is necessary. Findings that raise concern for ischemia include: mural thickening with a target or double halo sign; hyperdense attenuation in the bowel wall on non-contrast CT from intra-mural hemorrhage; bowel dilatation; pneumatosis; pneumoperitoneum; and mesenteric or portal venous gas. The most specific sign for ischemia is lack of bowel wall enhancement. There may be edema or hemorrhage in the small bowel mesentery or pericolonic fat.

Management

Management is generally conservative with bowel rest, IV fluids, and broad-spectrum antibiotics. More than 85 percent patients improve in just a few days. Surgery is indicated if there is clinical evidence of peritonitis or perforation.

Further Reading

1. Elder K, Lashner BA, Solaiman FA. Clinical approach to colonic ischemia. *Cleve Clin J Med* 2009; 76:401–409.

History

▸ 56-year-old man with decreased stool caliber and abdominal fullness.

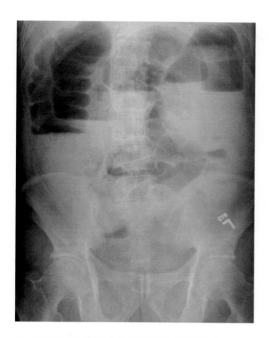

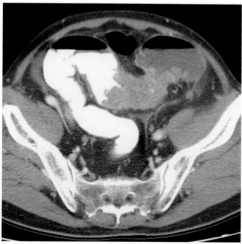

Case 68 Sigmoid Colon Cancer with Colonic Obstruction

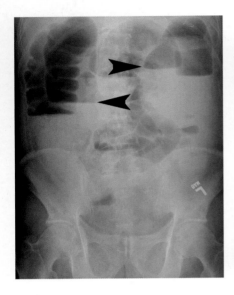 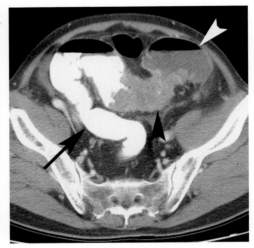

Findings

Upright abdomen radiograph (left) shows multiple air and fluid levels (arrowheads) within a dilated colon, indicating colonic obstruction. CT (right) shows dense rectal contrast (black arrow) that fills the sigmoid but does not pass a circumferential colonic mass (black arrowhead). Descending colon dilatation (white arrowhead) is seen proximal to the mass.

Differential Diagnosis

► Diverticulitis: may show focal colonic wall thickening, but usually associated with diverticulosis and signs of sepsis with acute symptoms. Lymphadenopathy is uncommon.
► Colonic metastasis: history of other malignancy.

Teaching Points

Left-sided and sigmoid colon adenocarcinomas are much more common than right-sided colon cancers. Typical clinical symptoms of left-sided cancers include reduction in stool caliber, bright red blood per rectum, and colonic obstruction. Due to the larger caliber of and the more liquid consistency of stool in the right colon, findings of anemia and weight loss are more common with right than with left colon cancers. The differentiation of perforated colon cancer from diverticulitis is occasionally ambiguous at CT, but colon cancer typically involves a more focal area of bowel and is more frequently associated with lymphadenopathy than diverticulitis. Of note, colon cancer may be associated with upstream or downstream colonic wall thickening, which may mimic a primary inflammatory rather than malignant process. For definitive diagnosis, colonoscopy may be required after acute symptoms resolve.

Management

Evaluation for local and distant metastases is critical for staging. Chemoradiation therapy is usually performed prior to surgical resection. However, if colonic obstruction is present, surgery may be required prior to other treatment.

Further Reading

1. Sai VF, Velayos F, Neuhaus J, Westphalen AC. Colonoscopy after CT diagnosis of diverticulitis to exclude colon cancer: a systematic literature review. *Radiology*. 2012; *263*(2):383–390.

History

► 58-year-old man with right lower quadrant pain.

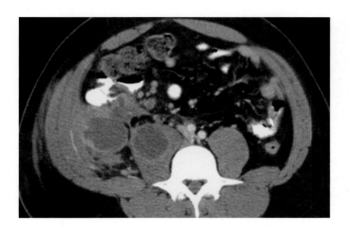

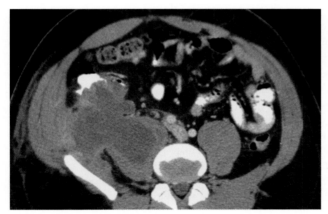

Case 69 Perforated Cecal Adenocarcinoma

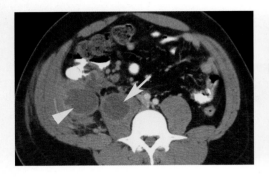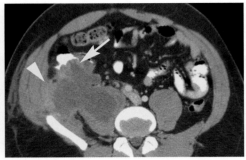

Findings

CT images show a large low-attenuation, rim-enhancing fluid collection extending from the posterior wall of the cecum into the psoas muscle (arrow in left image), pericecal fat (arrowhead in left image) and right lateral abdominal wall (arrowhead in right image). There is a polypoid mass along the posterior aspect of the cecal wall that extends into the cecal lumen (arrow in right image).

Differential Diagnosis

▶ Perforated inflammatory disorders of the ileocecal region such as appendicitis, cecal diverticulitis, and Crohn disease may be difficult to distinguish from perforated carcinoma, especially when there is a large abscess and marked inflammatory change. Features of each disorder should be sought out. For example, associated diverticula, an inflamed appendix, or findings that would suggest Crohn disease.

Teaching Points

Perforation is one of the major complications of colorectal adenocarcinoma. Other complications include bleeding and bowel obstruction. Perforations may result in abscesses, fistulas to adjacent organs such as the bladder, stomach, and adjacent segments of bowel, pneumoperitoneum, or pneumoretroperitoneum. Perforated carcinomas may be difficult to distinguish from diverticulitis with perforation. Observation of the following features may be helpful to favor carcinoma over diverticulitis: asymmetric wall thickening of the colon, soft tissue mass-like thickening of the colon wall, or the presence of an intraluminal polypoid mass. Inflammatory stranding, lymphadenopathy, and pericolonic fluid may be present in both conditions.

Management

The management of perforated colon cancer may include diverting colostomy with partial or complete colectomy performed at a single operation or over multiple operations. Percutaneous drainage of the abscess and endoscopic stenting of the colon are adjunctive or alternative options depending upon clinical condition of the patient.

Further Readings

1. Kobayashi H, Sakurai Y, Shoji M, et al. Psoas abscess and cellulitis of the right gluteal region resulting from carcinoma of the cecum. *J Gastroenterol.* 2001;36(9):623–628.
2. Maglinte DD, Pollack HM. Retroperitoneal abscess: a presentation of colon carcinoma. *Gastrointest Radiol.* 1983;8(2):177–181.

History

▸ 55-year-old man with abdominal distention.

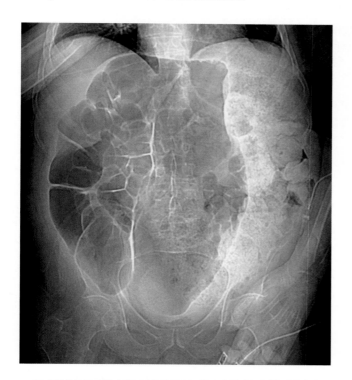

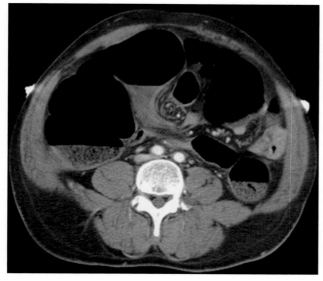

Case 70 Sigmoid Volvulus

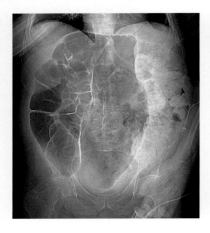 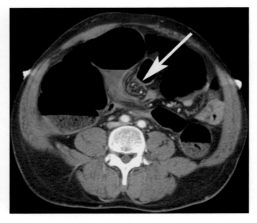

Findings

CT scout (left) reveals a dilated vertically orientated bowel loop in the mid abdomen with an "inverted U" or "coffee bean" configuration and absent haustra. CT (right) shows a "whirl sign" in the sigmoid colon mesentery (arrow) at the point of transition from dilated loops to decompressed colon.

Differential Diagnosis

► Cecal volvulus: the dilated loop of colon directed toward left upper abdomen, often with only one air-fluid level. The dilated cecum may have a "reverse C" configuration.
► Pseudo-obstruction: Massive colonic dilatation without obstruction. Rectal gas is usually seen, particularly on a right lateral decubitus or prone lateral view.
► Ileus: Dilated small and large bowel distended without a transition point.
► Large bowel obstruction due to other cause: dilated small bowel and colon proximal to the obstructing lesion.

Teaching Points

Sigmoid volvulus is the third leading cause of large bowel obstruction after diverticulitis and carcinoma in Western countries. In Western countries sigmoid volvulus is usually acquired from long-standing constipation, Parkinson disease, Alzheimer disease, or chronic debilitation. In other countries, Chagas disease and extreme high-fiber diet are causes. Radiographic findings include a "coffee bean" or "kidney bean" sign referring to a closed loop of sigmoid distended with gas, with apposed medial walls of dilated bowel forming an oblique line that resembles the cleft of a coffee bean. The dilated sigmoid classically points to right upper quadrant, but may be midline or leftward. On contrast enema, the twist in the bowel has a bird's beak appearance. The CT "whirl" sign, which is a visible twisting of both bowel and mesenteric vessels by over 180 degrees, is a known sign of volvulus but is nonspecific. Moderate or severe dilatation of the sigmoid with a sigmoid transition point is a more specific finding.

Management

Endoscopic or fluoroscopic decompression by barium enema is indicated if there are no contraindicating signs of bowel ischemia or perforation. Immediate surgical resection is performed when there is evidence of ischemia, perforation, or if decompression is unsuccessful.

Further Reading

Levsky JM, Den EI, DuBrow RA, Wolf EL, Rozenblit AM. CT findings of Sigmoid Volvulus. *Am J Roentgenol.* 2010; *194*: 136–143.

History

▶ 45-year-old man with HIV with intermittent bright red blood per rectum and pain with defecation.

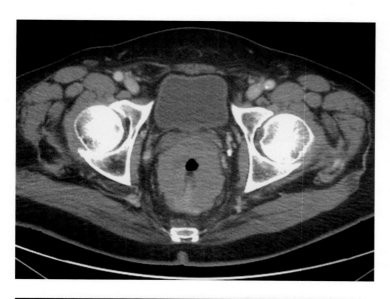

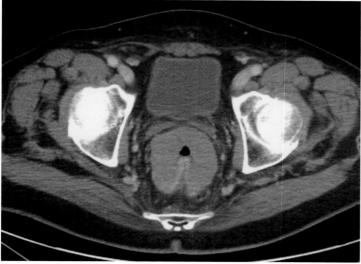

Case 71 Rectal Lymphoma in AIDS

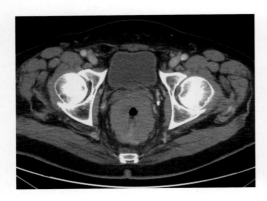 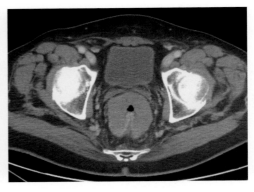

Findings

CT of the pelvis shows homogeneous attenuation and circumferential wall thickening of the rectum (up to 3 cm) with luminal narrowing.

Differential Diagnosis

► Rectal adenocarcinoma: may have similar findings on CT. Bowel obstruction and perforation occur much less often in patients with colorectal lymphoma than with colorectal adenocarcinoma.

► Edema from ischemia, inflammatory bowel disease, or infectious proctitis may cause circumferential wall thickening. The target sign of mucosal and muscularis propria hyperenhancement with hypoattenuating submucosal layer may help differentiate tumor from an inflammatory process on intravenous contrast-enhanced CT.

Teaching Points

Primary colorectal lymphoma is a rare type of gastrointestinal lymphoma and may be clinically indistinguishable from colorectal adenocarcinoma. Non-Hodgkin's lymphoma, usually of B-cell origin, comprises the majority of colorectal lymphomas. Patients with chronic immunosuppression, including patients with human immunodeficiency virus infection, are at increased risk for colorectal lymphoma. The signs and symptoms are relatively nonspecific, including abdominal pain, weight loss and lower gastrointestinal bleeding. Morphologically, colorectal lymphomas may manifest as a polypoid mass, an annular and infiltrating lesion, or as diffuse, multifocal polyps. The latter pattern is often referred to as lymphomatous polyposis. Rarely the mass will obstruct the large bowel. Associated pelvic lymphadenopathy is common.

Management

The treatment of primary rectal lymphoma is often surgical resection followed by multiagent systemic chemotherapy.

Further Readings

1. Dionigi G, Annoni M, Rovera F, Boni L, Villa F, Castano P, Bianchi V, Dionigi R. Primary colorectal lymphomas: Review of the Literature. *Surg Oncol.* 2007; *16*:S169–S171.
2. Ghai S, Pattison J, Ghai S, et. al. Primary gastrointestinal lymphoma: spectrum of imaging findings with pathologic correlation. *RadioGraphics.* 2007; *27*:1371–1388.

History

▶ 42-year-old female patient with rectal bleeding.

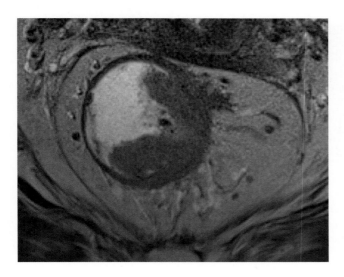

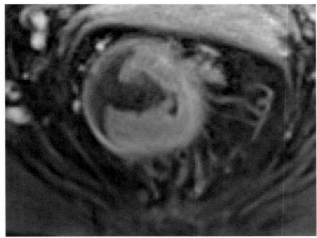

Case 72 Rectal Adenocarcinoma

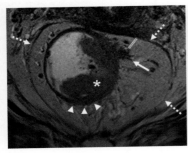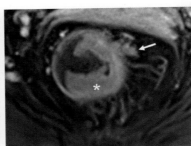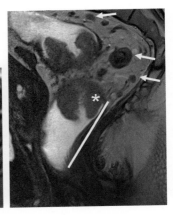

Findings

T2-weighted (left) and fat-suppressed enhanced T1-weighted (middle) MR images show an enhancing rectal tumor with a lobulated contour (asterisks). Tumor transgresses the muscularis propria (white arrowheads) and extends into the mesorectal fat (solid white arrow). The mesorectal fascia (dashed white arrows) is not involved. The circumferential resection margin (CRM) is 8 mm (double white line). Sagittal T2-weighted (right) image shows a distance of 4 cm from the inferior attachment of the rectal mass (asterisks) to the superior aspect of the anal sphincter (solid white line). Numerous lymph nodes with mixed signal intensity and ill-defined margins are present in the mesorectal fat (solid white arrows).

Differential Diagnosis

▶ Gastrointestinal stromal tumor: are submucosal lesions that often have a prominent extraluminal component. Lymphadenopathy is not a feature of these lesions.
▶ Lymphoma: anorectal lymphomas occur almost exclusively in the setting of AIDS. Lymphomas usually have minimal enhancement.
▶ Carcinoid: usually small submucosal masses of polyps when they arise in the rectum.

Teaching Points

On T2-weighted MR, the muscularis propria is the hypointense outer layer of the rectum, the inner mucosal/submucosal layer is hyperintense, and the surrounding mesorectal fat is hyperintense. The hypointense mesorectal fascia surrounds the mesorectal fat and is a natural plane for surgical resection. Rectal carcinoma has intermediate signal. MR diagnosis of TNM stage T2 tumors is characterized by involvement of the muscularis propria without extension through its outer border into the mesorectal fat. Stage T3 tumors disrupt the muscularis propria and extend into the mesorectal fat with a nodular or spiculated advancing margin. Tumor extension within 6 mm from the mesorectal fascia has been shown to be associated with a high risk of local recurrence. Mesorectal lymph nodes with irregular borders or mixed signal intensity are suspicious for harboring foci of carcinoma, especially when larger than 5 mm.

Management

MRI is helpful in staging to determine which patients will require preoperative neo-adjuvant chemoradiotherapy.

Further Reading

1. Iafrate F, Laghi A, Paolantonio P, et al. Preoperative staging of rectal cancer with MR imaging: Correlation with surgical and histopathologic findings. *RadioGraphics*. 2006; *26*: 701–714.

History

▶ 35-year-old man with rectal bleeding.

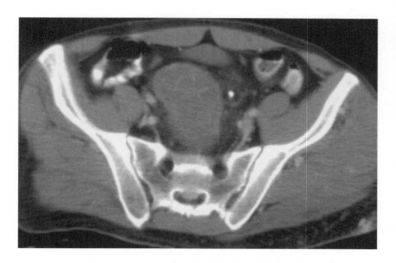

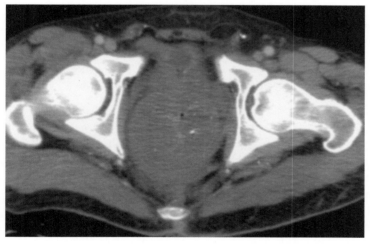

Case 73 Rectal Hemangioma

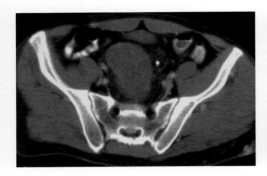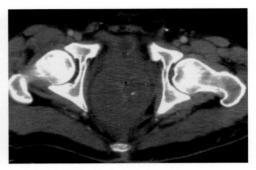

Findings

CT scan shows circumferential thickening of the rectum with luminal narrowing. Punctate rounded calcifications are present in the rectal wall thickening (left) and in the perirectal fat (right)

Differential Diagnosis

► Rectal adenocarcinoma: focal cancers may present with similar rectal wall thickening and associated luminal narrowing. Calcification may occur in mucinous tumors in a dot and dash configuration. Rectal carcinoma is more likely to demonstrate invasion with extension beyond the rectal wall and perirectal lymphadenopathy.

► Rectal lymphoma: patients with chronic immunosuppression are at increased risk for colorectal lymphoma. Circumferential wall thickening with luminal narrowing are common findings. Calcification is uncommon.

► Inflammatory and infectious rectal wall thickening: may have a similar appearance. The presence of a target sign on intravenous contrast-enhanced CT is a helpful finding to suggest an inflammatory etiology of rectal wall thickening.

Teaching Points

Colorectal hemangiomas are rare benign lesions that are a potential source of significant lower-gastrointestinal bleeding. The rectosigmoid is the most common site of colonic hemangiomas. They commonly affect younger adults and are occasionally associated with Klippel-Trenaunay-Weber syndrome, Maffucci syndrome, blue rubber bleb nevus syndrome, and diffuse neonatal hemangiomatosis. Clinically, patients may present with acute, recurrent, or chronic painless rectal bleeding. CT may demonstrate a thickened rectosigmoid and pelvic phleboliths within the hemangioma and mesenteric veins. Enhancement with intravenous contrast may be seen and the mesenteric vasculature may be engorged. Serpentine borders and the presence of phleboliths are helpful distinguishing features.

Management

Surgical resection is the definitive therapy. For nonsurgical candidates, alternate therapies reported in the literature include sclerotherapy, polypectomy, electrocautery, angiographic embolization, and irradiation.

Further Reading

1. Levy AD, Abbott RM, Rohrmann CA, et al. Gastrointestinal hemangiomas: imaging findings with pathologic correlation in pediatric and adult patients. *Am J Roentgenol.* 2001; *177*(5): 1073–1081.

History

▶ 42-year-old man with intermittent diarrhea, occasionally bloody, for 10 to 15 years. Patient has a family history of colon carcinoma.

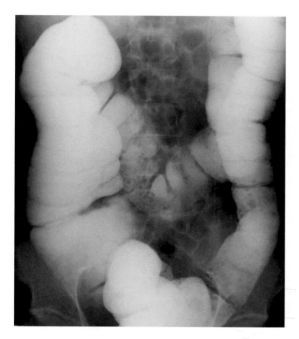

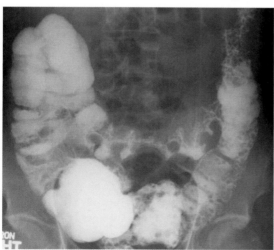

Case 74 Familial Adenomatous Polyposis Syndrome (FAP)

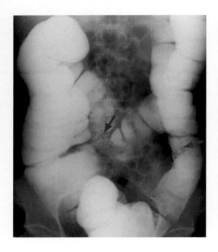 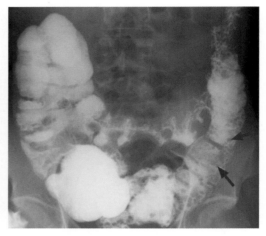

Findings

Barium enema shows innumerable small, round filling defects (arrows) within the colon secondary to multiple polyps.

Differential Diagnosis

▶ Retained feces: fecal matter may be distinguished by different projections demonstrating non-adherence to bowel wall.

▶ Inflammatory pseudopolyps: patients with inflammatory bowel disease can have islands of elevated, inflamed tissue surrounded by ulceration mimicking a polyp. Patient history usually will help with diagnosis.

▶ Lymphoid hyperplasia: can be seen in up to 50 percent of pediatric barium studies and 13 percent of adults. This will appear as innumerable tiny filling defects distributed in a generalized pattern in the small bowel and colon ,which is unlike the distribution of familial adenomatous polyposis where nodules more concentrated on colon; particularly in the rectosigmoid region.

Teaching Points

Familial adenomatous polyposis is an autosomal dominant disease caused by a germline abnormality of the adenomatous polyposis coli gene on the long arm of chromosome 5. Familial adenomatous polyposis is characterized by the presence of hundreds or thousands of colorectal adenomatous polyps with near 100 percent malignant transformation by age 40. Polyps typically begin to develop at the onset of puberty and become symptomatic with rectal bleeding and diarrhea in 75 percent of cases. Familial adenomatous polyposis has equal distribution in both male and female patients and is estimated to affect 1 in 10,000 people in the United States. Gardner's Syndrome is a variant of familial adenomatous polyposis with extra-intestinal findings of abdominal desmoid tumors, mandibular osteomas and epidermoid cysts. Turcot syndrome is another familial adenomatous polyposis variant with increased incidence of central nervous system medulloblastoma and malignant gliomas.

Management

Treatment consists of a prophylactic procto-colectomy when the patient is approximately 20 years of age, with an ileo-anal anastomosis.

Further Reading

1. Rusti, AK . Hereditary gastrointestinal polyposis and non-polyposis syndromes. *N Engl J Med*. 1994:*331*(25)1694–1702.

History

▸ 68-year-old man with right lower quadrant pain and fever.

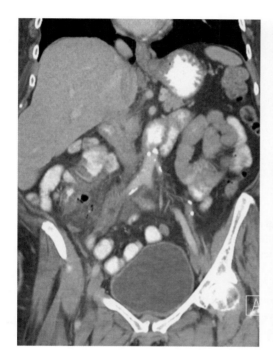
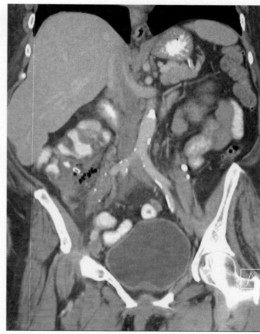

Case 75 Cecal Diverticulitis

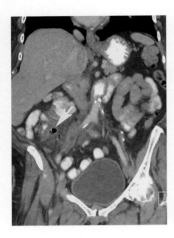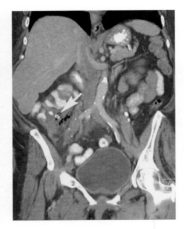

Findings

CT (left image) shows a diverticulum (arrow) on the medial aspect of the cecum surrounded by fat stranding and foci of extraluminal air with associated colonic wall thickening. A more posterior image (right image) shows a fecalith (arrows). The appendix is normal (not shown).

Differential Diagnosis

► Perforated colon carcinoma: may be difficult to distinguish from cecal diverticulitis. Enhancing asymmetric soft tissue thickening or mass of the cecal wall is suggestive of carcinoma, particularly when associated with lymphadenopathy.

► Appendicitis: with perforation and abscess formation may be indistinguishable from cecal diverticulitis. The location of the epicenter of the inflammation may be suggestive if the appendix is not visualized.

► Inflammatory disease of the terminal ileum: such as Crohn disease, should be considered if there is terminal ileum and other noncontiguous segments of bowel involvement.

Teaching Points

Cecal diverticula may be congenital or acquired. Congenital diverticula are composed of all three layers of the bowel wall. They are uncommon and are typically solitary and larger than the more common acquired diverticula. Acquired diverticula are mucosal herniations through the colon wall and are typically multiple, small. The findings of cecal diverticulitis are similar to sigmoid diverticulitis: pericolonic soft tissue stranding and fluid, fascial thickening, symmetric thickening of the cecal wall, diverticula, and in more severe cases, intramural or pericolonic abscesses. Cecal diverticulitis with abscess may be difficult to differentiate from perforated appendicitis. The location of the inflammatory process downstream to the base of the cecum and the presence of adjacent cecal diverticula are suggestive of diverticulitis.

Management

Patients with mild diverticulitis with or without a small abscess are usually treated conservatively with antibiotics and bowel rest. Percutaneous catheter drainage and antibiotics are used to treat patients with large abscesses. Elective surgical resection is performed later for these patients. Immediate surgery is usually reserved for patients with free perforation and peritonitis.

Further Reading

1. Jang HJ, Lim HK, Lee SJ, Lee WJ, Kim EY, Kim SH. Acute diverticulitis of the cecum and ascending colon: the value of thin-section helical CT findings in excluding colonic carcinoma. *Am J Roentgenol.* 2000;*174*(5):1397–1402.

History

► 45-year-old woman with pelvic pain.

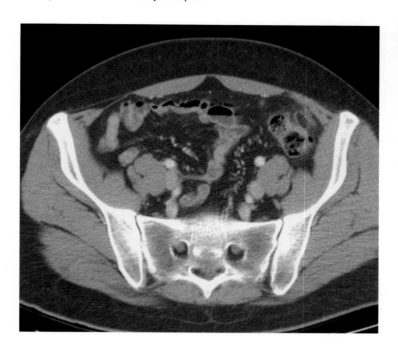

Case 76 Epiploic appendagitis

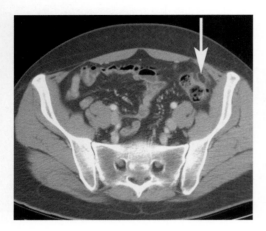

Findings

CT shows an oval-shaped fatty mass (arrow) with a thin enhancing rim in the sigmoid mesocolon surrounded by fat stranding (ring sign). A faint central engorged vessel (central dot) is seen within the fatty mass. No colonic wall thickening is present.

Differential Diagnosis

► Omental torsion and infarction: tends to be larger and more circular in shape. A swirl in the omentum may be seen from the torsion.
► Diverticulitis: presence of an inflamed diverticulum and tends to have thickening of the involved segment of colon, pericolonic inflammatory change and fluid.
► Mesenteric panniculitis: most commonly located at the root of the small bowel mesentery. The fat surrounding the mesenteric vessels may be preserved (the *fat ring sign*).

Teaching Points

Epiploic appendages are peritoneal outpouchings that arise from the serosal surface of the colon and contain fat and blood vessels. Idiopathic inflammation is proposed to be a result of torsion or occlusion of a central draining vein. There is controversy about the role of predisposing factors such as obesity and heavy exercise. The clinical symptoms may mimic diverticulitis if in the left lower quadrant and appendicitis if in the right lower quadrant. CT findings include a 1.5 to 3.5 cm diameter round or oval fat attenuation lesion with surrounding inflammatory change adjacent to the antimesenteric colonic wall. Colonic wall thickening and or peritoneal thickening can be present, but the colonic wall thickening tends to be mild. A central high-density focus is thought to represent the thrombosed vessel. This "central dot" sign is diagnostic when present, but its absence does not preclude a diagnosis of epiploic appendagitis. The peripheral rim of the fatty mass is inflammatory thickening of the parietal peritoneum. Over time, findings may remain the same, or the size of lesion may decrease with minimal or no residual soft tissue attenuation.

Management

Epiploic appendagitis is a benign, self-limited disease. Treatment is conservative with pain medication.

Further Reading

1. Singh AK, Gervais DA, Hahn PF, Rhea J, Mueller PR. CT appearance of Acute Appendagitis. *Am J Roentgenol.* 2004; *183*:1303–1307.

History

▶ 50-year-old woman with pelvic pressure and low back pain. Pelvic MRI is performed for evaluation.

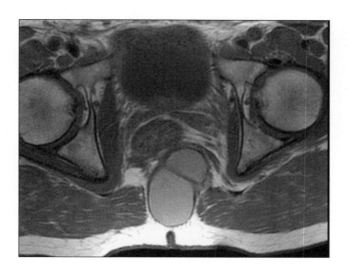

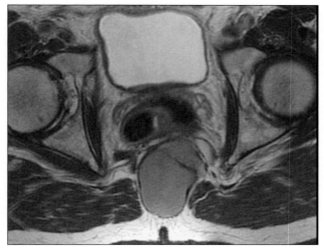

Case 77   Tail Gut Cyst

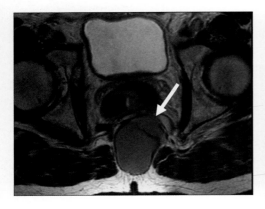 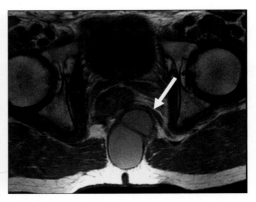

Findings

Axial images from T2-weighted (left) and T1-weighted (right) MRI sequences show a unilocular, thin-walled, presacral cyst with a thin internal septation and internal content that is intermediate signal intensity on both sequences (arrow). No mural soft tissue nodules are present.

Differential Diagnosis

► Sacrococcygeal teratoma: typically heterogeneous, solid, and partly cystic presacral masses, often with calcifications or fat. Rarely, these are entirely cystic. They are uncommonly diagnosed in adults.
► Anterior sacral meningocele: would communicate with the subarachnoid space through a sacral defect.
► Pyogenic abscess: would usually present with surrounding inflammatory changes and symptoms referable to a pelvic infection.

Teaching Points

Dermoid cysts, neurenteric cysts, epidermoid cysts, and enteric cysts are the four types of congenital, epithelial-lined, retrorectal developmental cysts that occur in the presacral space. When diagnosed in adult women, these cysts are often asymptomatic. Enteric cysts have two forms: tailgut cysts and cystic rectal duplication. Tailgut cysts are remnants of the embryologic hindgut and are also referred to as retrorectal cystic hamartomas. Unlike true duplication cysts, which are lined by mucin-secreting columnar cells and have submucosa and muscularis propria similar to the normal gastrointestinal wall, tailgut cysts may have various epithelial linings (mucin-secreting columnar, transitional, and squamous) and lack the well developed mural layers of a duplication cyst. When clinically symptomatic, tailgut cysts cause symptoms related to mass effect or complications from fistualization, superimposed hemorrhage, or malignant degeneration. By imaging, tailgut cysts are well circumscribed, thin walled, uni- or multilocular lesions with proteinaceous internal content that often is intermediate to hyperintense on T1WI. Thin internal septations may be seen. Soft tissue mural nodularity may correlate with malignant degeneration. Rarely, mural calcification may be seen.

Management

Tailgut cysts are treated with surgical resection to confirm the diagnosis and frequently to cure.

Further Reading
1. Yang DM, Park CH, Jin W, et al. Tailgut cyst: MRI evaluation. *Am J Roentgenol.* 2005;*184*(5):1519–1523.

History

▶ 61-year-old man with several hours of increasing abdominal pain and distension.

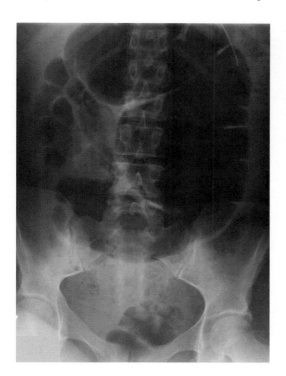

Case 78   Cecal Volvulus

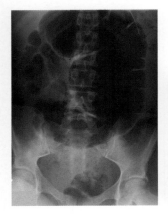 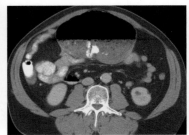 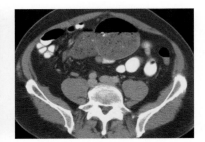

Findings

Supine radiograph (left) shows a distended upturned cecum with the configuration of a reversed letter C. There is gas-filled small bowel, paucity of gas in the ascending colon, and gas in the rectum. Complementary CT shows malposition of the cecum to the midline, swirl of the mesentery, and beak-like tapering of the twisted cecum.

Differential Diagnosis

▶ Sigmoid volvulus: the classic radiographic appearance consists of a dilated segment of sigmoid that has an inverted U configuration, with its apex in the right upper quadrant, midline, or left upper quadrant. The inner walls of the sigmoid may oppose one another, producing a central line that points toward the pelvis and a configuration often referred to as the "coffee bean sign." The distended sigmoid may also elevate the diaphragm. CT reveals the sigmoid as the involved segment of bowel with swirling of the sigmoid mesentery.

▶ Large bowel obstruction secondary to tumor, hernia or intussusception: radiographs show a large bowel obstruction. CT will often be useful in differentiating between these etiologies and cecal volvulus.

Teaching Points

Volvulus is twisting of the bowel around its own mesentery that often results in a partial or complete closed-loop obstruction. Cecal volvulus is less common and occurs in slightly younger patients than sigmoid volvulus; it accounts for 25 to 40 percent of cases of volvulus of the colon and about 1 percent of intestinal obstruction. Inadequate fixation and persistence of an ascending colon mesentery, or incomplete embryologic rotation of the bowel, results in a freely mobile cecum and an increased risk for cecal volvulus formation. Typically, patients develop sudden onset of abdominal pain and distention. Less commonly, patients may present with more chronic abdominal symptoms. Early diagnosis is of utmost importance because a delay in diagnosis increases the risk of vascular compromise and subsequent bowel necrosis.

Management

Emergent detorsion with a colonoscopy may be performed. However, in general, the treatment for cecal volvulus is surgery.

Further Reading

1. Moore C, Corl F, Fishman E. CT of cecal volvulus: unraveling the image. *Am J Roentgenol.* 2001; *177*(1):95–98.

Part 7 Liver

History

▶ 59-year-old man with left-sided abdominal pain and an incidental finding in the liver.

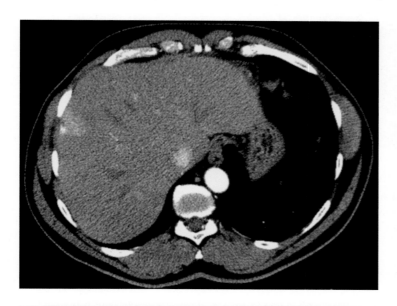

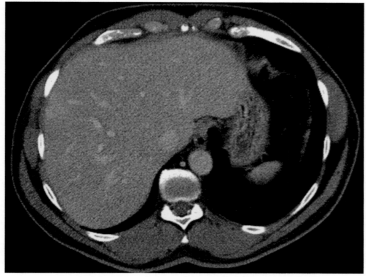

Case 79 Transient Hepatic Attenuation Difference (THAD)

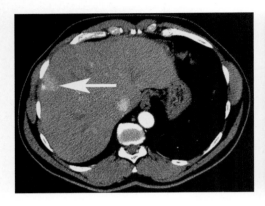 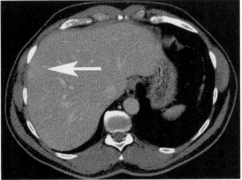

Findings

CT obtained during the arterial phase (left image) shows a focal, peripheral, wedge-shaped area of hyperenhancement (arrow). No associated mass is visible. Portal venous phase image (right) shows near disappearance of the abnormality, with only vague residual hyperenhancement (arrow).

Differential Diagnosis

▶ Hepatocellular carcinoma: mass-like arterial phase hyperenhancement with hypoenhancement on venous or delayed phases (washout).
▶ Hypervascular liver metastasis: typically mass-like, but may be associated with perfusion abnormality due to vascular shunt or occlusion of adjacent portal vein.
▶ Focal nodular hyperplasia: arterial phase hyperenhancement with later phase isoenhancement and delayed enhancement of a central scar.

Teaching Points

Transient hepatic attenuation differences (THADs) are small, triangular or geographic, subsegmental foci of arterial phase hepatic hyperenhancement that typically extend to the liver capsule and disappear during other phases of liver enhancement. They are most commonly idiopathic but can be secondary to an adjacent mass (benign or malignant), trauma, biopsy, portal venous branch thrombosis, or to "siphoning" from an adjacent inflammatory process. The benign form should be distinguished from a perfusion abnormality secondary to an adjacent mass at the apex of the abnormality. In cirrhosis, care should be taken to distinguish THADs from hepatocellular carcinoma, which characteristically demonstrates mass-like arterial enhancement with washout and/or interval growth. Transient hepatic intensity differences (THIDs) are the contrast-enhanced MR imaging equivalents of THADs.

Management

Careful inspection of THADs should be done to exclude an underlying mass. THADs with an identifiable cause (e.g. metastasis, benign mass, pyogenic abscess, trauma) should be managed accordingly.

Further Readings

1. Kim H, Kim A, Kim T, et. al. Transient Hepatic Attenuation Differences in Focal Hepatic Lesions: Dynamic CT features. *Am J Roentgenol.* 2005;*184*:83–90.
2. Colagrande S, Centi N, Galdiero R, Ragozzino A. Transient Hepatic Intensity Differences: Part 1, Those Associated with Focal Lesions. *Am J Roentgenol.* 2007;*188*:154–159.
3. Colagrande S, Centi N, Galdiero R, Ragozzino A. Transient Hepatic Intensity Differences: Part 2, Those Not Associated with Focal Lesions. *Am J Roentgenol.* 2007;*188*:160–166.

History

► 60-year-old man referred to MR imaging.

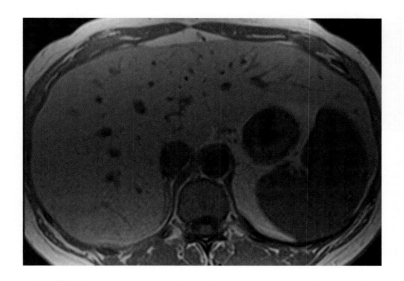

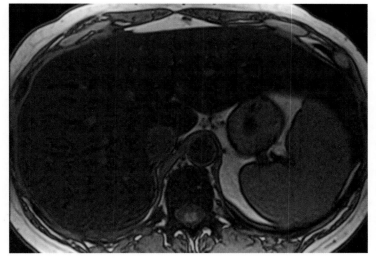

Case 80 Hepatic Steatosis

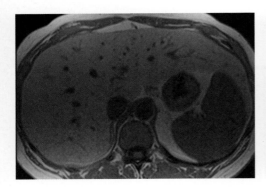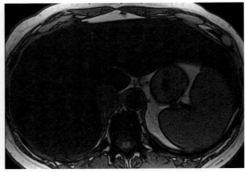

Findings

T1-weighted gradient echo in-phase image (left) shows higher hepatic signal intensity relative to that of the spleen. On the T1-weighted gradient echo out-of-phase image (right), there is significant drop of signal in the liver relative to the spleen, indicative for intravoxel fat.

Differential Diagnosis

▶ Steatohepatitis: biopsy is needed to distinguish steatosis from steatohepatitis, which may be associated with hepatic enlargement.

▶ Hemosiderosis or hemochromatosis: increased hepatic parenchymal signal (rather than decreased) on out-of-phase phase gradient echo T1-weighted MR images which have a shorter TE at 1.5 tesla compared to in-phase images, and therefore less susceptibility artifacts.

Teaching Points

Hepatic steatosis is a common condition, historically associated with alcohol use, diabetes, obesity, and certain drugs. Idiopathic hepatic steatosis is called non-alcoholic fatty liver disease (NAFLD) and predicts insulin resistance and metabolic X syndrome. Hepatic steatosis is epidemic, with steatosis now seen in up to 33 percent of the general population. Most patients are asymptomatic, but the condition can progress to steatohepatitis and cirrhosis and increase the risk for hepatocellular carcinoma. On gradient echo MR images, hepatic steatosis is characterized by focal or diffuse loss of hepatic T1 signal intensity relative to spleen on opposed-phase compared to in-phase images. At unenhanced CT, liver attenuation more than 10 Hounsfield units less than spleen suggests steatosis. Because of aberrant blood supply, focal deposition commonly occurs around the falciform ligament, fissure for the ligamentum teres hepatis, and adjacent to the gallbladder fossa. Vessels that course though the abnormality suggest fatty change rather than a true mass.

Management

Management of hepatic steatosis focuses on removing or controlling any identifiable offending agents. Abstinence from alcohol can reverse the process in alcoholic forms. Control of diabetes, weight management, and control of hyperlipidemia can be effective in slowing the disease process. Some patients may progress to steatohepatitis and cirrhosis.

Further Reading

1. Ma X, Holalkere N, Kambadakone A, Mino-Kenudson M, Hahn P, Sahani D. Imaging-based Quantification of Hepatic Fat: Methods and Clinical Applications. *RadioGraphics*. 2009; *29*:1253–1277.

History

► 55-year-old man with elevated liver function tests.

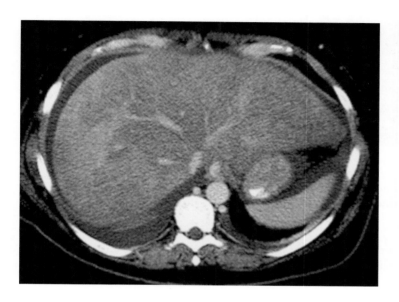

Case 81   Focal Steatosis

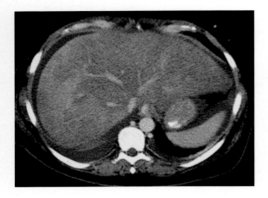

Findings

CT shows heterogeneous enhancement with patchy, geographic low attenuation areas. Vessels coursing through the regions of low attenuation areas are nondisplaced.

Differential Diagnosis

► Masses such as hepatocellular adenoma, angiomyolipoma, and myelolipomas: may have foci of macroscopic fat seen but will have mass effect and spherical contour.

Teaching Points

Steatosis, or fatty liver, is a reversible accumulation of triglycerides in the hepatocytes due to toxic, ischemic, or infectious insults. Involvement can be uniform, patchy, focal, or, rarely, periportal and subcapsular. Focal deposition occurs in typical areas that include the medial segments of the left lobe, adjacent to the falciform ligament, anterior to the porta hepatis, and adjacent to the gallbladder fossa. Patchy deposition may be related to regional differences or disturbances in hepatic blood flow from aberrant veins that enter the liver independently from the portal venous system, including cholecystic veins, and other peribiliary veins. Other causes include high triglyceride levels, chemotherapy, alcohol abuse, diabetes mellitus, obesity, exogenous steroids, and parenteral nutrition. Steatosis is diagnosed on unenhanced CT images when the liver attenuation is 10 Hounsfield units lower than that of the spleen. Usually focal areas are well defined, wedge-shaped areas with geographic borders. Occasionally, focal fat can have a nodular or segmental distribution and mimic malignant disease, particularly hepatocellular carcinoma or hepatic adenomas, which are tumors that occasionally have fatty components. The diagnosis of focal steatosis is suggested by lack of mass effect on vessels and ducts that traverse the focal steatotic areas, and lack of the typical arterial hypervascularity and capsule that is commonly seen with tumors. MRI gradient echo and out-of-phase T1 weighted sequences are diagnostic; the fatty areas lose signal on out-of-phase images indicating the presence of microscopic fat.

Management

No management is necessary. Focal steatosis may resolve if the inciting toxin or alcohol is removed.

Further Reading

1. Yoshimitsu K, Honda H, Kuroiwa T, Irie H, Aibe H, Shinozaki K, Masuda K. Unusual hemodynamics and pseudolesions of the noncirrhotic liver at CT. *RadioGraphics*. 2001; *21*: S81–S96.

History

▸ 58-year-old man with alcoholism and hepatitis C.

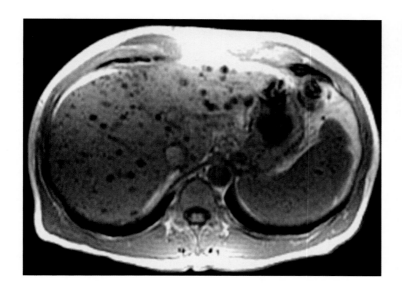

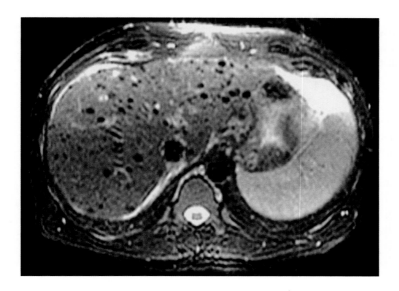

Case 82 Cirrhosis

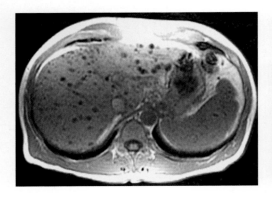 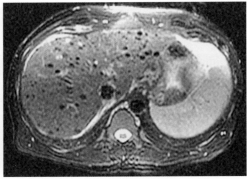

Findings

Axial T1- (left) and T2-weighted (right) MR images show a liver with nodular contour and multiple small siderotic regenerative nodules which are hypointense on both images due to paramagnetic effect of iron. A few hypointense siderotic nodules are also seen in the spleen, where they are known as Gamna-Gandy bodies.

Differential Diagnosis

▶ Treated hepatic metastases or lymphoma: usually has a history of extrahepatic malignancy. Treated metastatic breast cancer may simulate the radiologic appearance of cirrhosis ("pseudo-cirrhosis").

▶ Budd-Chiari syndrome (hepatic venous outflow obstruction): may show caudate hypertrophy, heterogeneously diminished enhancement in the liver periphery, ascites and splenomegaly. Absence of patent hepatic veins suggests the diagnosis.

▶ Hepatic sarcoidosis: Hypointense hepatic and splenic nodules are seen on T1 and T2 weighted MR along with hepatosplenomegally and adenopathy. Differentiate by looking for other imaging and clinical findings of sarcoidosis.

Teaching Points

The leading causes of cirrhosis in the United States are hepatitis C, hepatitis B, and alcohol consumption. Chronic hepatocyte injury results in inflammation, fibrosis, and regenerative nodules. Patients with cirrhosis are at risk for developing life threatening hepatocellular carcinoma (HCC). Many types of regenerative nodules have been described. Siderotic (iron-containing) nodules are generally benign, but benign regenerative nodules may progress to dysplastic nodules to hepatocellular carcinoma. Tiny (less than 1 cm) hypervascular nodules that are not seen on other phases of enhancement are generally benign, but should be followed closely by imaging to exclude malignancy. Hepatic fibrosis causes portal hypertension with associated imaging findings including portosystemic shunts, ascites, and splenomegaly.

Management

Patients with cirrhosis have a 1 to 4 percent annual risk of developing hepatocellular carcinoma and therefore need regular screening. The ideal screening method (ultrasound, CT, MRI, and/or alpha-fetoprotein) has not been established, but it is believed that screening for hepatocellular carcinoma reduces mortality in high-risk patients.

Further Readings

1. Brancatelli G, Federle MP, Ambrosini R, et al. Cirrhosis: CT and MR imaging evaluation. *Eur J Radiol*. 2007; *61*(1): 57–69.
2. Hussain SM, Reinhold C, Mitchell DG. Cirrhosis and lesion characterization at MR imaging. *RadioGraphics*. 2009; *29*: 1637–1652.

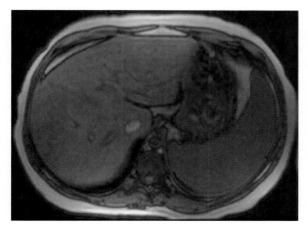

History

▶ 10-year-old boy presenting with jaundice and elevated blood glucose.

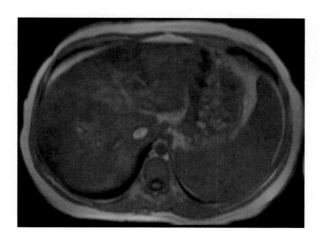

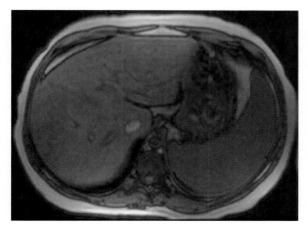

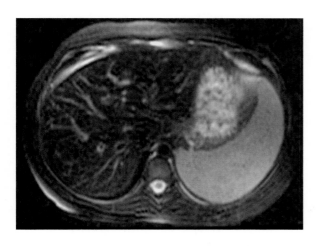

Case 83 Primary Hemochromatosis

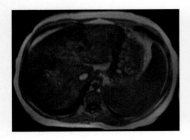
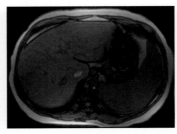
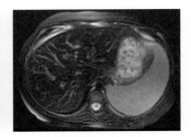

Findings

Transverse gradient echo T1-weighted in-phase image (left) obtained with a TE of 2.1 msec shows diffusely lower signal in the liver than on the opposed phase (center) image which was obtained with a longer TE of 4.2 msec. This is the opposite of the finding seen with diffuse hepatic steatosis. T2-weighted fat saturation image (right) shows marked diffuse hypointensity of the liver. Splenomegaly suggests portal hypertension

Differential Diagnosis

▶ None: these findings are specific for hepatic iron storage disease.

Teaching Points

Primary hemochromatosis is caused by an autosomal recessive disorder of iron absorption resulting in excess iron deposition in many tissues including liver, pancreas, and heart. Secondary hemochromatosis is an acquired disease with multiple etiologies including chronic transfusion and myelodysplastic syndrome. In the secondary form of the disease, iron deposition is seen primarily in the reticuloendothelial system, so it can often be differentiated from primary disease by noting involvement of the spleen and bone marrow; however there is overlap in the imaging features between the primary and secondary forms. Owing to magnetic field inhomogeneities caused by iron deposition, characteristic local reductions of MR signal are seen for sequences with longer echo times, including T2*- and T2-weighted sequences and in-phase images compared with opposed-phase images that are acquired with shorter echo times.

Management

Gradient echo and T2* weighted imaging can be used to identify and estimate the degree of iron deposition in the liver noninvasively. Iron overload may be treated with phlebotomy or iron chelation therapy.

Further Readings

1. Merkle EM, and Rendon CN. Dual gradient-echo in-phase and opposed-phase hepatic MR imaging: a useful tool for evaluating more than fatty infiltration or fatty sparing. *RadioGraphics.* 2006; *26*: 1409–1418.
2. Queiroz-Andrade M, et al. MR imaging findings of iron overload. *RadioGraphics* 2009; *29*: 1575–1589.

History

▶ 41-year-old man with end-stage renal disease and status post renal transplant.

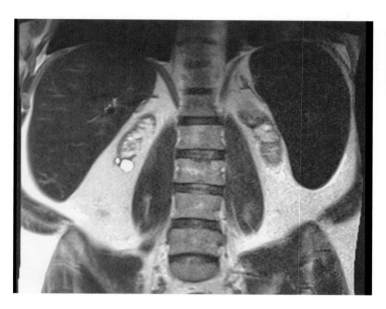

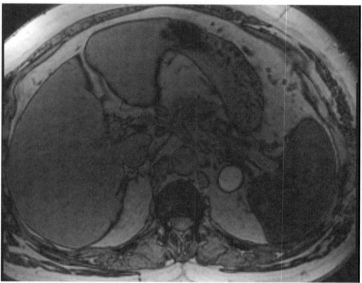

Case 84 Hemosiderosis

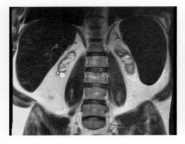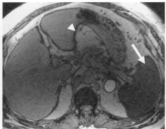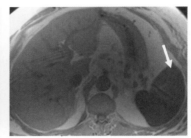

Findings

T2-weighted MR (left) shows abnormal low signal intensity liver, and especially the and spleen. Out-of-phase gradient-echo T1-weighted image (middle) shows the typical chemical shift artifact (arrowhead) of an out of phase image and unusual low signal intensity of the spleen. On the in-phase gradient-echo T1-weighted image (right), obtained with a longer echo time, there is shows further decrease of the signal intensity of the spleen (arrow), and to a lesser extent the liver. In iron storage disease, the parenchymal signal intensity decreases on the image with the longer echo time due to the continued decay of the transverse magnetization.

Differential Diagnosis

▶ Hereditary hemochromatosis: excess iron is stored in hepatocytes, not in the reticuloendothelial system. Therefore, the spleen is normal signal intensity in patients with hemochromatosis.

Teaching Points

In patients with hemosiderosis or siderosis, either due to transfusional iron overload states or dyserythropoiesis (e.g. thalassemia major, sideroblastic anemia, pyruvate kinase deficiency, chronic liver disease), the excessive iron is processed and accumulates in organs containing reticuloendothelial cells, including liver, spleen, and bone marrow. The superparamagnetic effect of accumulated iron in the Kupffer cells results in significant reduction of signal intensity of the liver parenchyma on T2-WI. T2*-weighted and other gradient-echo sequences are the most sensitive to magnetic susceptibility effects of ferritin and hemosiderin because of their lack of a 180-degree refocusing pulse. Comparison of the signal intensity of liver with that of paraspinal muscles, which are normally less intense than liver and not prone to excessive iron accumulation, provides a useful internal control: if the signal intensity of liver is less (on all sequences) than that of paraspinal muscle, it should be considered abnormal.

Management

Although in general the clinical significance of transfusional iron overload states is negligible, patients undergoing chronic transfusion can develop "secondary" hemochromatosis characterized by progressive liver dysfunction due to saturation of their reticuloendothelial system.

Further Reading

1. Mortele KJ, Ros PR. Imaging of diffuse liver disease. *Semin Liver Dis.* 2001;*21*:195–212.

History

► 56-year-old man with heart disease and elevated liver enzymes for 20 years.

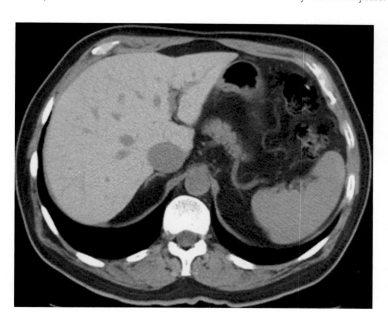

Case 85 Amiodarone Deposition

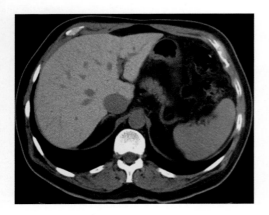

Findings

Unenhanced CT image through the upper abdomen demonstrates diffuse high CT attenuation of the liver relative to the spleen. No focal lesions are present.

Differential Diagnosis

▶ Hemochromatosis: in primary hemochromatosis, an iron overload disorder, the liver, pancreas, and heart can be involved. Late stage shows cirrhotic features.

▶ Hemosiderosis: iron accumulation in the reticuloendothelial system that includes the liver, spleen, lymph nodes, and bone marrow; no organ damage. Typically due to extensive blood transfusions.

▶ Wilson disease: copper deposition in the liver leads to cirrhosis, usually causes fat depositon and does not increase liver attenuation; hyperdense regenerating nodules can be seen.

▶ Glycogen storage disease: can be associated with hepatic adenomas.

Teaching Points

Amiodarone is an iodinated drug used to treat refractory supraventricular and ventricular arrhythmias. Amiodarone and its metabolite desethylamiodarone may be stored in the liver causing liver damage ranging from mild reversible injury to acute liver failure and irreversible cirrhosis. On unenhanced CT, the CT number of the liver may be as high as 95 to 145 Hounsfield units (normal 45 to 65HU), due to the high concentrations of the iodinated drug and its metabolite. By comparison, the hepatic and portal veins appear hypodense relative to the parenchyma but are normal in CT number. Pulmonary fibrosis is also a well known complication. Findings in the lung on a high resolution CT include diffuse interstitial and interlobular septal thickening, chronic organizing pneumonia (formerly known as bronchiolitis obliterans organizing pneumonia), or dependent consolidations. Often the area of involved lung shows high attenuation as well.

Management

Elevated hepatic enzymes and CT attenuation of the liver can normalize after cessation of amiodarone intake. Nonalcoholic steatohepatitis and cirrhosis can occur with long-term amiodarone administration. Monitoring liver function and/or liver biopsy is recommended before irreversible damage is reached.

Further Reading

1. Goldman IS, Winkler ML, Raper SE, et al. Increased hepatic density and phospholipidosis due to amiodarone. *Am J Roentgenol.* 1985; *144*(3):541–546.

History

▶ 83-year-old woman with long-standing heart disease.

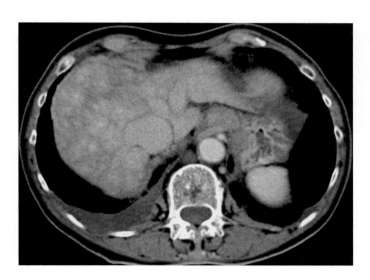

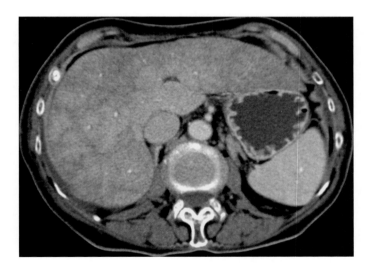

Case 86 Passive Hepatic Congestion

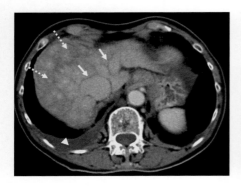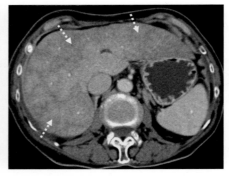

Findings

Portal venous phase CT shows early retrograde filling of distended hepatic veins and IVC (solid arrows), and heterogeneous mottled hepatic parenchymal enhancement (dashed arrows). There is a small right pleural effusion (arrowhead).

Differential Diagnosis

► Budd-Chiari syndrome: characterized by narrowed or obstructed inferior vena cava or hepatic veins. "Flip-flop" enhancement pattern occurs in which the central liver enhances normally in contrast to the periphery of the liver. In later phases of enhancement, the central portions of the liver wash out and there is delayed enhancement of the periphery.

► Hepatic veno-occlusive disease: narrowed, but patent, hepatic veins that may occur four to five weeks after hematopoietic stem cell transplantation, radiation therapy, chemotherapy, or ingestion of "bush tea".

► Acute hepatitis: normal caliber hepatic and portal veins with normal vascular pattern. Hepatomegaly is usually present and the parenchymal enhancement pattern is normal.

Teaching Points

Passive hepatic congestion occurs when there is stasis of blood within the liver parenchyma as a result of impaired venous drainage in patients with poor right heart function from congestive heart failure, constrictive pericarditis, cardiomyopathies, right-sided valvular disease, or pericardial effusion. The incidence and prevalence is unknown. Patients may present with right upper quadrant pain, hepatomegaly, elevated liver function tests, ascites, or jaundice.

On CT, early enhancement of a dilated IVC and central hepatic veins occurs from reflux of contrast from the right ventricle. During the portal venous phase, the liver has a heterogeneous, mottled, or reticulated pattern of parenchymal enhancement. Along the periphery of the liver, slow or stagnant flow results in patchy areas of poor or delayed enhancement. Perivascular lymphedema may also be seen as linear low attenuation surrounding the portal veins and intrahepatic IVC, which should not be confused with venous thrombosis. Secondary CT findings that suggest the diagnosis include hepatomegaly, ascites, periportal and gallbladder wall edema, cardiomegaly, and pleural or pericardial effusions.

Management

Managing the cause of the elevated right heart pressures can lead to full recovery if hepatic fibrosis has not occurred.

Further Reading

1. Gore RM, Mathieu DG, White EM, et al. Passive hepatic congestion: cross-sectional imaging features. *Am J Roentgenol.* 1994;*162*:71–75.

History

▶ 48-year-old female patient with newly diagnosed soft tissue sarcoma arising from the left calf. CT scan was performed for staging.

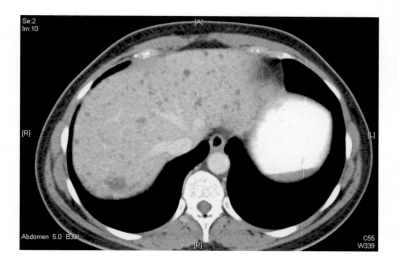

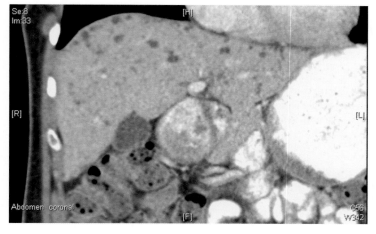

Case 87 Biliary Hamartomas

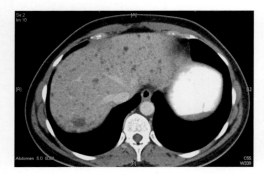 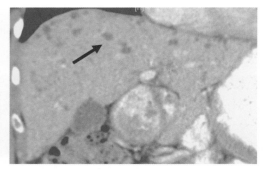

Findings

Axial (left) and coronal (right) intravenous contrast-enhanced CT images obtained during the portal venous phase demonstrate innumerable hypodense lesions that are scattered throughout the liver parenchyma. No perceptible enhancement of the lesions is noted. All lesions measure less than 1.5 cm in size and have an irregular contour (arrow).

Differential Diagnosis

▸ Hepatic microabscesses: most common in immunocompromised patients and demonstrate peripheral rim-like enhancement.
▸ Diffuse liver metastases: typically have intermediate attenuation and less well-defined margins.
▸ Hepatic (bile duct cysts): typically round or oval in shape, have a smooth contour, and are variable in size, frequently measuring larger than 1.5 cm.

Teaching Points

Biliary hamartomas, also called von Meyenburg complexes, are thought to result from embryonic bile ducts (ductal plate) that fail to develop normally, and are considered part of the congenital hepatic fibropolycystic disease spectrum. Therefore, they may coexist with other hepatic manifestations, such as Caroli disease or hepatic fibrosis. Biliary hamartomas are generally asymptomatic and are usually encountered as an incidental finding at imaging, laparotomy, or autopsy. On MR imaging, these foci appear as high signal on T2-weighted and low signal on T1-weighted images.

Management

If diagnosis is uncertain on sonography or CT scan, an MRI with T2-WI can be performed to confirm the cystic nature of the lesions. Biliary hamartomas are, in general, benign developmental lesions and therefore don't need any further follow-up or treatment.

Further Readings

1. Brancatelli G, et al. Fibropolycystic liver disease: CT and MR imaging findings. *RadioGraphics.* 2005;25:659–670.
2. Mortele KJ, et al. Cystic focal liver lesions in the adult: differential CT and MR imaging features. *RadioGraphics.* 2001;21:895–910.
3. Tohme-Noun C, Cazals et al. Multiple biliary hamartomas: magnetic resonance features with histopathologic correlation. *Eur Radiol.* 2008;18:493–499.

History

▶ 32-year-old woman with acute onset of jaundice, right upper quadrant pain, and abdominal distention.

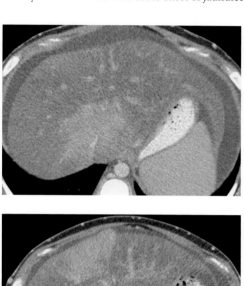

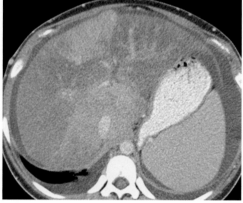

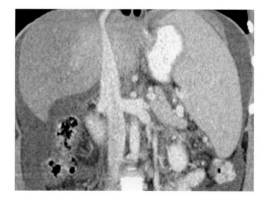

Case 88   Budd-Chiari Syndrome

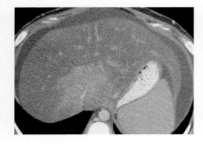 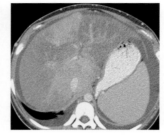 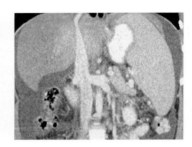

Findings

CT obtained in the portal venous phase shows moderate ascites, hepatomegaly, and heterogeneous liver enhancement with decreased peripheral perfusion. The central liver and caudate lobe enhance normally. The hepatic veins do not enhance and the IVC is narrowed. Also present are splenomegaly and superficial collateral veins in the anterior abdominal wall.

Differential Diagnosis

▶ Cirrhosis: atrophy of the right and medial segment of the left hepatic lobes. Portal hypertension can cause varices, ascites and splenomegaly, but the hepatic veins are normal in size and patent.
▶ Veno-occlusive disease: hepatomegaly, hepatic vein narrowing (rather than occlusion), periportal cuffing, gallbladder wall edema, and findings related to portal hypertension, including splenomegaly and ascites.
▶ Passive hepatic congestion: reflux of contrast from the right atrium into enlarged hepatic veins and IVC with a heterogeneous, mottled mosaic pattern of enhancement in the portal venous phase. Hepatomegaly and ascites may be present.

Teaching Points

Budd-Chiari syndrome is caused by hepatic venous outflow obstruction at the level of the hepatic veins or inferior vena cava. It may be primary or secondary. Primary causes include venous webs and diaphragms, injury, and infection. Secondary causes most commonly are thrombotic, related to hypercoaguable states or to chemotherapy and radiation. Budd-Chiari syndrome has variable imaging features, including hepatic vein or IVC thrombosis, changes in liver morphology and enhancement patterns, intrahepatic venous collaterals ("comma sign"), varices and ascites. In acute Budd-Chiari, the liver is globally enlarged and associated with congested peripheral regions, with decreased contrast enhancement and stronger enhancement in the central liver areas. After intravenous contrast administration, preserved enhancement is seen in areas of venous drainage that are less affected, such as the caudate lobe because of its direct venous outflow in the inferior vena cava.

Management

Anticoagulant therapy is used to prevent recurrence and extension of thrombosis, along with measures to control ascites and gastrointestinal bleeding. Portosystemic shunt (TIPS), cavoplasty, or liver transplantation may be necessary.

Further Reading

1. Torabi M, Hosseinzadeh K, Federle MP. CT of Nonneoplastic Hepatic Vascular and Perfusion Disorders. *RadioGraphics*. 2008;*28*:1967–1982.

History

► 48-year-old woman with abdominal mesenteric desmoid tumors and multiple hepatic lesions that have been stable for five years.

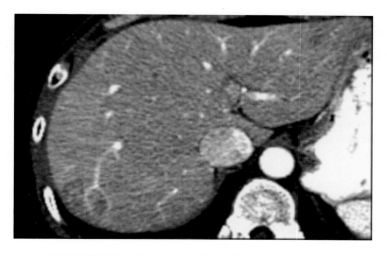

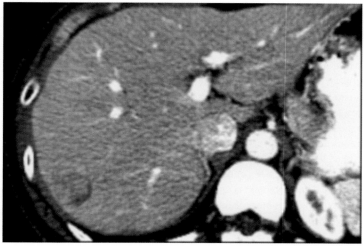

Case 89 Hepatic Peliosis

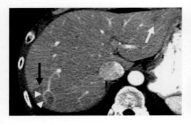 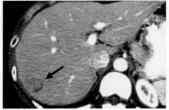 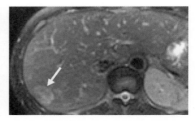

Findings

CT images obtained during the portal venous phase shows a partially enhancing focal hepatic lesion in the right lobe of the liver (black arrow). The lesion causes no mass affect on adjacent hepatic vessels (arrowheads). T2-weighted MR (right) shows hyperintense signal within the mass (arrow).

Differential Diagnosis

- ► Hemangioma: peripheral, nodular and discontinuous enhancement, which parallels the blood pool.
- ► Focal nodular hyperplasia: homogeneous enhancement on the arterial phase and isoattenuating on the portal venous and delayed phases. May have a central scar that shows delayed enhancement.
- ► Hepatic adenoma: may contain fat and adenomas are usually solitary (70 to 80 percent), unless associated with glycogen storage disease or liver adenomatosis.
- ► Hypervascular metastases/hepatocellular carcinoma: HCC usually has washout on the portal venous or delayed phase.

Teaching Points

Peliosis hepatis is a rare benign vascular lesion characterized by sinusoidal dilatation and blood-filled spaces. In 20 to 50 percent of cases, no associated condition is identified. Peliosis is caused by toxins (arsenic and polyvinyl chloride) and certain hepatotoxic drugs including oral contraceptives, anabolic steroids, corticosteroids, and chemotherapeutic agents. It may also occur because of disseminated tuberculosis and infection from *Bartonella* (bacillary peliosis) in AIDS. On unenhanced CT, hepatic peliosis is low attenuation. The size of lesions can vary and the lesions may contain thrombus, hemorrhage, and calcification. During the arterial phase of contrast enhancement, lesions typically have early globular enhancement, small accumulations of contrast material in the center (target sign), and no mass effect on surrounding hepatic vessels. In the portal venous phase, centrifugal enhancement is usually seen; however, centripetal progression has been described. Then, during the delayed phase, homogeneous hyperattenuation (blood pooling), can be seen. The MR signal intensity is variable. Most lesions are hyperintense on T2-weighted images.

Management

Peliosis hepatis may resolve after withdrawal of the offending drug or toxin. Antibiotic therapy can lead to clinical improvement in AIDS-related bacillary peliosis.

Further Reading

1. Iannaccone R, Federle MP, Brancatelli G, et al. Peliosis hepatis: spectrum of imaging findings. *Am J Roentgenol.* 2006; *187*:43–52.

History

► 37-year-old woman with right upper quadrant pain.

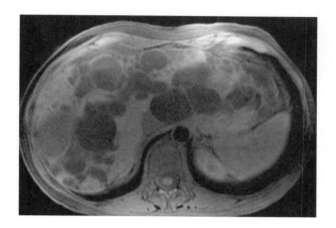

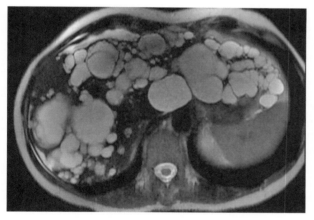

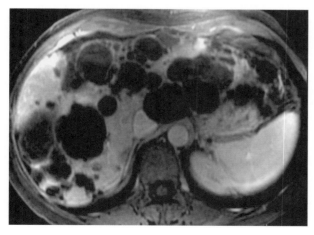

Case 90   Polycystic Liver Disease (PCLD)

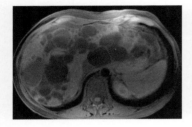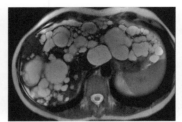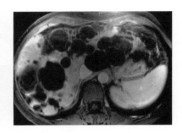

Findings

MR images of the liver show multiple cystic lesions in the liver that are hypointense relative to the hepatic parenchyma on T1 (left), hyperintense relative to hepatic parenchyma on T2 (middle) and do not have enhancement after contrast administration (right).

Differential Diagnosis

► Biliary hamartomas/von Meyenberg complexes: small, disconnected embryologic bile ducts, irregular in shape, and usually measure less than 15 mm in diameter. MR signal characteristics are the same as simple hepatic cysts.

► Simple hepatic (bile duct) cysts: usually measure between 1 and 5 cm and are more often multiple than solitary. If complicated by infection or hemorrhage they will have variable signal on T1- and T2-weighted imaging.

► Caroli disease: saccular or fusiform dilation of the intrahepatic bile ducts.

Teaching Points

Polycystic liver disease is characterised by variable replacement of hepatic parenchyma with multiple cysts. It is an autosomal dominant condition and is associated with autosomal dominant polycystic kidney disease (ADPKD). However, there is a much rarer form that arises separately from ADPKD and has an incidence of 0.02 percent. The majority of lesions are asymptomatic or may be associated with abdominal pain and early satiety from hepatomegaly, nausea, ascites, and dyspnea. Complications include cyst rupture, infection, or hemorrhage in the cyst. Polycystic liver disease may be classified into three types: type 1 has ≤10 large cysts with large area of normal liver parenchyma; type 2 has diffuse medium-sized cysts with remaining large areas of the normal liver parenchyma; and type 3 has massive diffuse mixed small- and medium-sized cysts with minimal normal intervening liver parenchyma. On MRI, the cysts are hypointense relative to hepatic parenchyma on T1, hyperintense relative to hepatic parenchyma on T2, and they do not enhance with intravenous contrast. If complicated by intra-cystic hemorrhage or infection, they may have variable signal intensity on both T1- and T2-weighted imaging.

Management

Surgical procedures such as cyst aspiration and sclerosis, open or laparoscopic cyst fenestration or marsupialisation, liver resection, or liver transplant are considered for symptomatic patients.

Further Reading

1. Morgan DE, Lockhart ME, Canon C, et al. Polycystic liver disease: Multimodality imaging for complications and transplant evaluation. *RadioGraphics*. 2006;*26*:1665–1668.

History

▶ 21-year-old woman with incidental liver mass detected at routine US evaluation. MRI is obtained for further characterization.

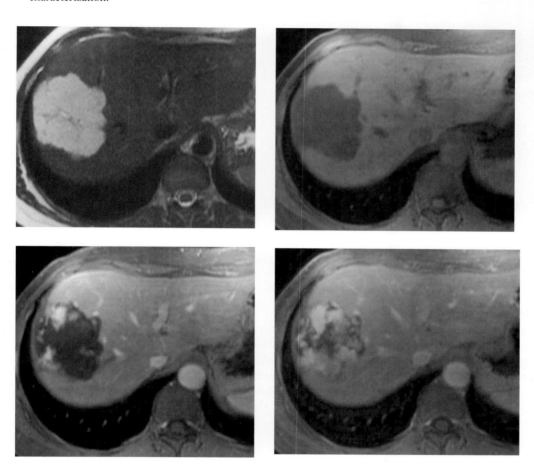

Case 91 Hepatic Cavernous Hemangioma

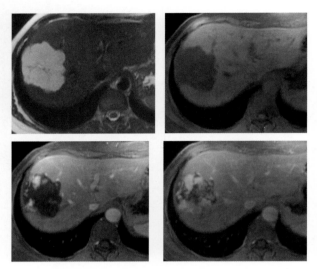

Findings

T2-weighted (upper left) and T1-weighted (upper right) images demonstrate a large mass with lobulated margins showing low signal intensity on T1 and very high signal on T2. Portal venous and delayed contrast-enhanced images (lower left and right) show gradual centripetal enhancement with peripheral, nodular, and discontinuous pattern in the portal venous phase. The areas of enhancement are isointense to blood pool.

Differential Diagnosis

▶ Peripheral (intrahepatic) cholangiocarcinoma: central delayed and persistent enhancement may mimic hemangioma. Cholangiocarcinoma is hypovascular, often heterogeneous and hypointense on T2. It may have capsular retraction, bile duct dilatation, and vascular invasion.
▶ Focal nodular hyperplasia: isodense or isointense to the surrounding liver parenchyma on precontrast and portal venous phase CT and MR images, with a T2 hyperintense central scar that enhances on delayed images.
▶ Hypervascular metastasis: usually multiple, but rarely may be as T2 bright as hemangiomas. Metastases are commonly hypointense or isointense on portal venous and delayed phases.

Teaching Points

Cavernous hemangiomas are the most common benign tumors of the liver. Imaging characteristics include a homogeneous and hyperechoic appearance on US, with posterior acoustic enhancement, though at times hemangiomas may be hypoechoic. At unenhanced CT and T1 weighted MR imaging, findings are hypodense and isointensity to liver parenchyma, respectively. Hemangiomas have sharply defined lobulated borders and very high signal on T2-weighted MR images. After contrast administration, the lesions show early nodular peripheral enhancement with progressive centripetal filling, though small hemangiomas may show flash filling such that they enhance homogeneously almost instantaneously. Hemangiomas may coexist with other tumors and are generally asymptomatic. Rarely, hemangiomas may be very large and cause symptoms related to mass effect or vascular shunting. Spontaneous rupture of a hepatic hemangioma is uncommon.

Management

Cavernous hemangiomas are benign and usually require no therapy. Large, symptomatic hemangiomas may necessitate surgery.

Further Reading

1. Silva AC, Evans JM, McCullough AE, et al. MR Imaging of Hypervascular Liver Masses: A Review of Current Techniques. *RadioGraphics*. 2009;29:385–402

History

▶ 66-year-old asymptomatic woman with incidentally discovered liver mass.

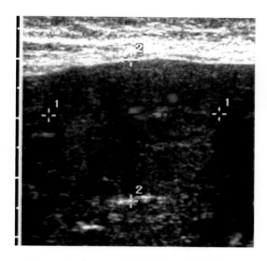

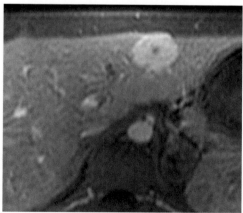

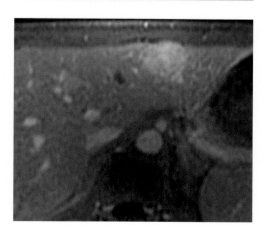

Case 92   Focal Nodular Hyperplasia

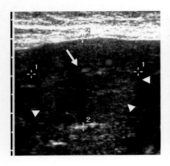 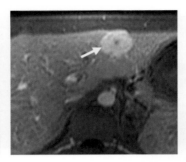 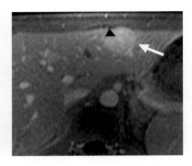

Findings

Ultrasound (left) shows a mildly hyperechoic mass in the liver (arrowheads) with central regions of vascularity (white arrow). Gadolinium-enhanced T1-weighted images show early intense homogeneous enhancement of the mass (white arrow on middle image). Portal venous phase (right) shows delayed enhancement of the central scar (black arrowhead).

Differential Diagnosis

► Fibrolamellar hepatocellular carcinoma: central scar can calcify in 55 percent of cases and demonstrates hypointensity on T2-weighted images and no delayed hyperenhancement. Internal hemorrhage and necrosis cause heterogeneous signal intensity.

► Hepatocellular adenoma: may have internal hemorrhage. It usually does not have a central scar and is often encapsulated.

► Hepatocellular carcinoma: delayed contrast-enhanced images show internal washout and tumor capsule may be seen. Vascular invasion, metastasis, and lymphadenopathy may be present.

Teaching Points

Focal nodular hyperplasia (FNH) occurs most commonly in women. Generally, FNH is a solitary, nonencapsulated, well circumscribed and lobulated mass that contains a central scar. On US, FNH usually appears as a homogenous iso- or slightly hypoechoic mass. The central scar is often difficult to visualize with US, however when seen is usually hyperechoic and hypervascular with Doppler US. On CT, FNH is iso- to slightly hypoattenuating mass with contrast. During the arterial phase of enhancement, FNH shows immediate and intense enhancement (with exception of the central scar) becoming isodense to the liver during the portal venous phase. The central scar enhances on the delayed phase. Typical MR features of FNH are iso- or hypointensity on T1 weighted images and slight homogenous hyper- or isointensity on T2. The central scar is hyperintense on T2-WI because of the presence of water-rich loose myxomatous fibrous tissue. The MR enhancement pattern is identical to CT.

Management

Hepatocyte-specific contrast agents or sulfur-colloid nuclear scintigraphy may be helpful to differentiate FNH from other lesions when there are atypical imaging features.

Further Reading

1. Mortele KJ, Praet M, Van Vlierberghe H, et al. CT and MR imaging findings in focal nodular hyperplasia of the liver: radiologic-pathologic correlation. *Am J Roentgenol.* 2000; *175*: 687–692.

History

▶ 42-year-old asymptomatic woman evaluated with MRI for incidentally detected liver lesion.

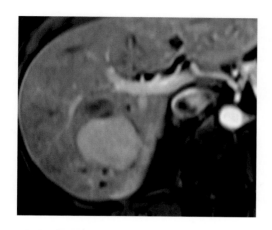

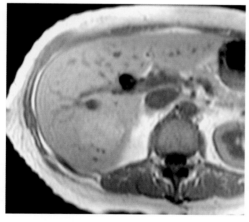

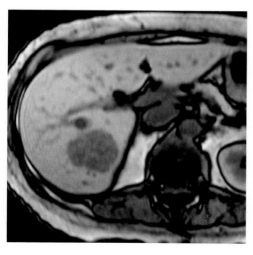

Case 93 Hepatocellular Adenoma

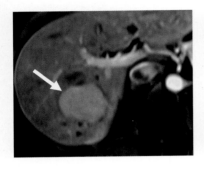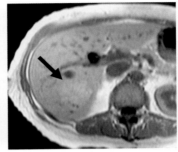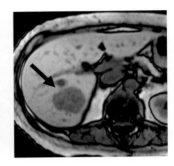

Findings

T1-weighted enhanced image (left image) shows a well-circumscribed homogeneously avidly enhancing mass (arrow) in the right lobe of a non-cirrhotic liver. Opposed phase T-1 weighted image shows loss of signal within the mass (arrow on right image) compared to the T1-weighted in-phase image (arrow on middle image).

Differential Diagnosis

► Focal nodular hyperplasia: does not typically contain lipid or hemorrhage. Homogeneous and lobulated mass with a central scar, which classically shows delayed enhancement.

► Fibrolamellar carcinoma: usually large and lobulated with heterogeneous enhancement. May have a central or eccentric scar, which does not usually enhance. Calcifications may occur in the scar.

► Hepatocellular carcinoma: most often occurs in cirrhotic liver and may contain fat. In some cases may be indistinguishable from hepatocellular adenoma.

► Hypervascular metastases: most are multiple and hypointense on T1-WI and markedly hyperintense on T2-WI. Fat and hemorrhage are rare.

Teaching Points

Hepatocellular adenoma is an uncommon benign hepatocellular neoplasm that most often occurs in young to middle-aged women with a history of oral contraceptive use. These lesions are typically solitary, but it is not unusual to see two or three in one patient. Multiple lesions can be seen in patients with glycogen storage disease and hepatocellular adenomatosis. Most patients with solitary adenomas are asymptomatic; however, large adenomas may cause right upper quadrant fullness or discomfort. Adenomas are sharply marginated, non-lobulated masses that may have a capsule. On MR, most adenomas are hyperintense on T1 due to increased glycogen, fat, and hemorrhage. When lipid is present in an adenoma, there is signal dropout on opposed-phase T1-weighted images. On T2, adenomas are predominantly hyperintense relative to liver; however. some can be hypo- or isointense. Most adenomas are heterogeneous on both T1 and T2 due to hemorrhage and necrosis. On gadolinium-enhanced sequences, hepatic adenomas have early arterial enhancement.

Management

Hepatocellular adenomas have a risk of hemorrhage and malignant transformation. Treatment strategies may vary from hormone therapy cessation, serial imaging to resection and embolization.

Further Reading

1. Grazioli L, Federle MP, Brancatelli G, et al. Hepatic adenomas: imaging and pathologic findings. *RadioGraphics*. 2001; *21*: 877–894.

History

▶ 44-year-old woman with primary sclerosing cholangitis.

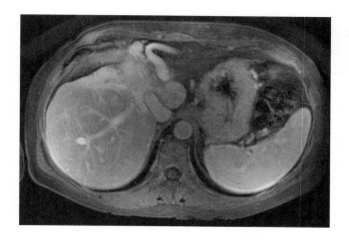

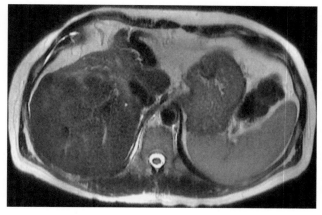

Case 94 Confluent Hepatic Fibrosis

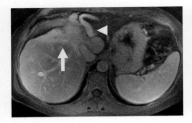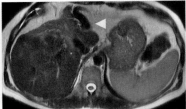

Findings

T1-weighted image obtained during delayed venous phase (left) of contrast enhancement shows capsular retraction at the level of the left medial segment and a peripheral wedge-shaped area of delayed parenchymal enhancement (long arrow) that is slightly hyperintense on the T2-weighted image (right). Vessels and bile ducts run through this area. An enlarged paraumbilical vein (arrowhead) is present in keeping with portal hypertension.

Differential Diagnosis

► Intrahepatic cholangiocarcinoma: may exhibit capsular retraction and delayed enhancement due to intratumoral fibrosis, but is frequently centrally T2 hypointense and associated with peripheral biliary duct dilatation. Satellite metastases also may be present.
► Cavernous hemangioma: may fibrose causing capsular retraction, particularly in cirrhotic livers. Hemangiomas are markedly T2 hyperintense, typically exhibit discontinuous, progressive, peripheral, nodular contrast enhancement. and lack associated biliary obstruction.
► Hepatocellular carcinoma: moderately T2 hyperintense with early arterial enhancement and tumoral washout on delayed phase imaging. Hepatocellular carcinoma usually lacks capsular retraction and may have mass effect on adjacent structures.

Teaching Points

Confluent hepatic fibrosis develops in the setting of cirrhosis, particularly in primary sclerosing cholangitis, and typically presents as a wedge-shaped area of parenchymal volume loss radiating from the hilum that generally involves the medial segment of the left lobe and/or the anterior segment of the right lobe. The involved liver is typically hypoattenuating and hypointense on unenhanced CT and T1-weighted MR imaging respectively, hypovascular during arterial and early venous post-contrast enhanced phases, and hyperintense on T2-weighted MR imaging. The T2 hyperintensity is likely from superimposed inflammation. Delayed enhancement of the fibrotic parenchyma is often seen. Although some imaging features of confluent hepatic fibrosis overlap with those of malignant neoplasms, confluent hepatic fibrosis typically does not show vascular displacement, portal venous washout, capsular bulge, or biliary obstruction.

Management

Biopsy or close imaging follow-up may be warranted if the characteristic imaging features are absent or the patient lacks the diagnosis of cirrhosis.

Further Reading

1. Ohtomo K, Baron RL, Dodd GD, et al. Confluent hepatic fibrosis in advanced cirrhosis: appearance at CT. *Radiology*. 1993;*188*(1):31–35.

History

▶ 52-year-old woman with intermittently elevated liver function tests.

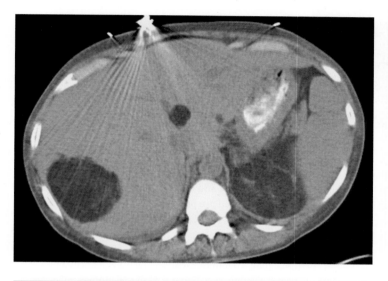

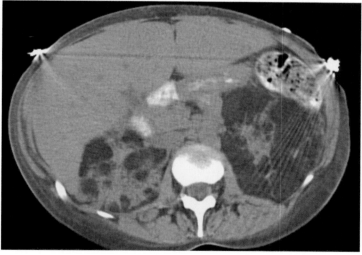

Case 95 Hepatic Angiomyolipoma in Tuberous Sclerosis Complex

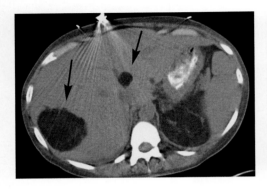 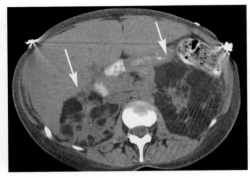

Findings

Axial MDCT images obtained with oral contrast and no intravenous contrast show two fat attenuation masses within the liver (black arrows). The larger is in the right hepatic lobe and the smaller in the medial segment of the left hepatic lobe. A few linear strands of soft tissue attenuation are present with the larger mass. Both kidneys (white arrows) are enlarged by innumerable fat-containing masses.

Differential Diagnosis

► Hepatocellular carcinoma and hepatocellular adenoma: may contain macroscopic fat. The majority of hepatocellular carcinomas occur in the setting of chronic liver disease. Hepatocellular adenomas may also have evidence of intratumoral hemorrhage and most commonly occur in women taking oral contraceptives.
► Metastatic liposarcoma: liver metastases occur in 10 percent of patients with liposarcoma.
► Myelolipoma: rarely occurs in the liver, indistinguishable from hepatic angiomyolipoma.

Teaching Points

Hepatic angiomyolipomas (AMLs) are benign, encapsulated mesenchymal tumors that histologically contain smooth muscle, thick-walled blood vessels, and mature adipose tissue. The majority of hepatic angiomyolipomas occur sporadically in general population. Six percent occur in patients with tuberous sclerosis complex. In patients with tuberous sclerosis complex, other stigmata of the disease such as renal angiomyolipomas may be present. Most patients are asymptomatic; however, spontaneous hemorrhage may occur and cause pain. The amount of fat within the lesion is variable. The fat component is echogenic on sonography and fat attenuation on CT. The fatty areas of AML may be interdigitated with vascular malformations and tissue showing early heterogeneous arterial enhancement, whereas the fat in fat-containing hepatocellular carcinoma is typically poorly enhancing.

Management

The majority of hepatic angiomyolipomas are asymptomatic and often are found incidentally. Because these lesions have no risk of malignant degeneration, surgery is reserved for those patients that have symptoms.

Further Reading

1. Basaran C, Karcaaltincaba M, Akata D, et al. Fat-containing lesions of the liver: cross-sectional imaging findings with emphasis on MRI. *Am J Roentgenol.* 2005;*184*(4):1103–1110.

History

► 50-year-old man with cirrhosis and hepatitis C.

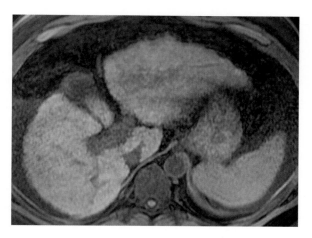

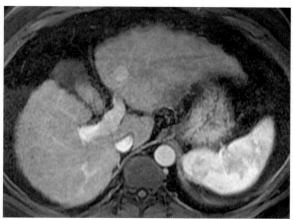

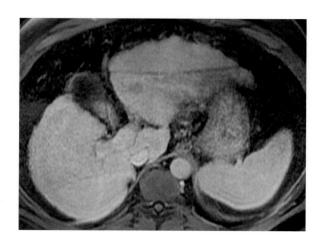

Case 96   Hepatocellular Carcinoma

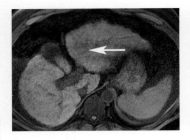 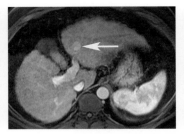 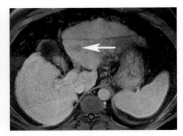

Findings

Gradient echo T1-weighted fat saturation pre-gadolinium axial image (left image) shows a faint mass (arrow) in a cirrhotic liver. This mass shows hyperenhancement on the late arterial phase (middle image) and hypoenhancement relative to liver parenchyma on the delayed phase (right image).

Differential Diagnosis

▶ Transient hepatic intensity difference (THID): isointense to liver on portal venous and delayed phases.
▶ Focal nodular hyperplasia (FNH): is typically isointense on portal venous and delayed phases with a late-enhancing scar.
▶ Hemangioma: The intensity of enhancement follows that of the blood pool, without delayed-phase washout.
▶ Intrahepatic cholangiocarcinoma: typically shows progressive delayed enhancement and is often associated with capsular retraction and bile duct dilatation.

Teaching Points

The finding of a mass with arterial phase hyperenhancement and either later-phase hypoenhancement relative to liver (washout) or growth more than 1 cm in one year is sufficiently specific to be generally considered diagnostic for hepatocellular carcinoma without biopsy for lesions larger than 2 cm. Ancillary features that suggest malignancy include a pseudocapsule surrounding the mass; mild to moderate hyperintensity on T2-ighted images; and reduced diffusion on DWI. Detailed standardized diagnostic criteria for hepatocellular carcinoma by MRI and CT can be found at www.acr.org/li-rads. Close interval follow-up or hepatobiliary contrast agents may be helpful for further evaluation of equivocal cases. PET imaging may not show increased FDG-uptake in well or moderately differentiated hepatocellular carcinomas.

Management

Based on a combination of tumor staging and liver function, treatment options include curative resection or transplantation; radiofrequency, alcohol or cryo-ablation; and chemoembolization of extensive or unresectable tumors. Imaging is often obtained for restaging after interventions as patients not previously eligible for transplantation may become eligible after ablation.

Further Readings

1. Willatt JM, Hussain HK, Adusumilli S, Marrero JA. MR Imaging of hepatocellular carcinoma in the cirrhotic liver: challenges and controversies. *Radiology.* 2008; *247*: 311–330.
2. Hussain SM, Zondervan PE, IJzermans JNM, Schalm SW, de Man RA, Krestin GP. Benign versus malignant hepatic nodules: MR imaging findings with pathologic correlation. *RadioGraphics.* 2002; *22*: 1023–1036.

History

▶ 27-year-old man with palpable mass and right upper quadrant abdominal pain.

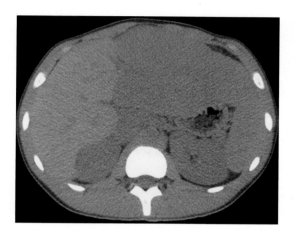

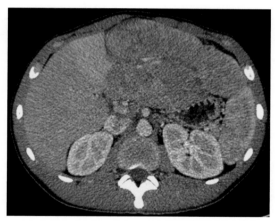

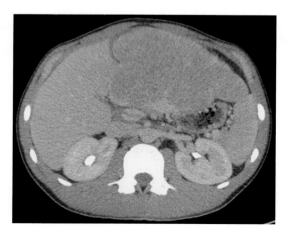

Case 97　Fibrolamellar Hepatocellular Carcinoma

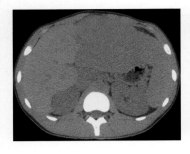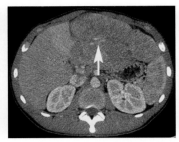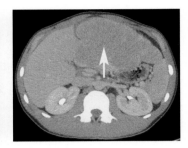

Findings

CT (left image) shows a large low-attenuation mass replacing the left lateral segment of the liver. CT in the arterial phase (middle image) shows heterogeneous enhancement of the mass with prominent vessels in a hypodense central scar (arrow). The delayed phase of enhancement (right image) shows hypoenhancement of the central scar (arrow).

Differential Diagnosis

▶ Hepatocellular carcinoma: may show central necrosis rather than a scar and usually occurs in the setting of cirrhosis or chronic liver disease.
▶ Focal nodular hyperplasia: homogeneous hypervascular arterial phase, isoattenuating on portal venous and delayed phases. Central scar enhances during the delayed phase.
▶ Hepatocelluar adenoma: may contain areas of necrosis, hemorrhage, or fibrosis that mimic a scar.
▶ Cavernous hemangioma: may contain central fibrosis that resembles a scar but the lesion continues to have the classic nodular discontinuous peripheral enhancement.

Teaching Points

Fibrolamellar hepatocellular carcinomas are rare, typically occurring in young adult patients without cirrhosis, chronic liver disease, or elevated tumor markers. The classic imaging appearance is a large, lobulated heterogeneous mass with a central scar in an otherwise normal liver. They are more commonly located in the left lobe of the liver than the right. Sonographically, the tumor demonstrates mixed echogenicity with a hyperechoic central scar. On CT, it is heterogeneous with areas of necrosis and hemorrhage. Approximately 40 percent of tumors have calcification in the central scar. The central scar is usually hypointense on T1- and T2-weighted sequences with absent or poor enhancement of the scar on delayed images. The scar can enhance on earlier phases if it has increased vascularity, cellularity, or myxomatous elements. Vascular invasion or multifocal disease is less commonly observed compared to conventional HCC.

Management

Surgical resection or liver transplant is the treatment for a large tumor. Five-year survival rate is approximately 67 percent, but the tumor frequently recurs.

Further Reading

1. Ichikawa T, Federle MP, Grazioli L, Madariaga J, Nalesnik M, Marsh W. Fibrolamellar hepatocellular carcinoma: imaging and pathologic findings in 31 recent cases. *Radiology*. 1999; *213*; 352–361.

History

▶ 66-year-old man with right upper quadrant abdominal pain.

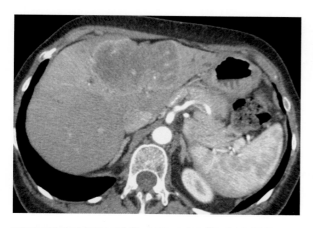

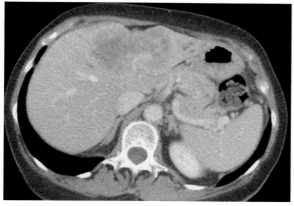

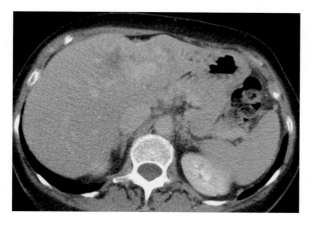

Case 98 Intrahepatic (Peripheral) Cholangiocarcinoma

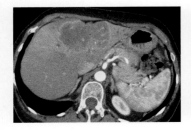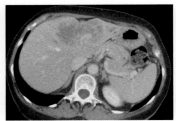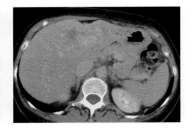

Findings

Late arterial phase (left), portal venous (middle), and delayed (right) phase contrast-enhanced CT images show an irregular large 10 cm solitary hepatic mass with associated capsular retraction and biliary dilatation in a noncirrhotic liver. There is thin irregular peripheral enhancement during the arterial and portal venous phases, along with central irregular prolonged enhancement on the delayed phase. No capsule, hemorrhage, or calcification is identified.

Differential Diagnosis

► Sclerosed hemangioma: usually shows typical peripheral interrupted nodular arterial enhancement that is isodense to the blood pool. The sclerosis may result in volume loss along with capsular retraction. No biliary dilation.

► Metastasis: often multiple. Rarely demonstrate capsular retraction, except in rare instances like treated breast metastasis.

► Hepatocellular carcinoma: arterial enhancement pattern with washout on delayed-phase images. Capsular retraction and biliary dilatation are uncommon.

► Confluent hepatic fibrosis: occurs in cirrhosis. It is often wedge-shaped and located within the anterior and medial segments of the liver, and usually has delayed enhancement on contrast-enhanced sequences.

Teaching Points

Intrahepatic (peripheral) cholangiocarcinoma is a primary adenocarcinoma that arises from the epithelium of small distal intrahepatic bile ducts beyond the secondary confluence. Intrahepatic cholangiocarcinoma may be associated with clonorchiasis, intrahepatic stone disease, Caroli disease, and primary sclerosing cholangitis. Peripheral cholangiocarcinomas classically present as large lobulated masses with capsular retraction and biliary dilatation. Satellite nodules are common. On arterial and portal venous contrast-enhanced CT, they demonstrate peripheral irregular enhancement that progresses to irregular central enhancement on delayed phases. Typical MR features are hypointensity on T1-weighted and central hypointensity on T2-weighted images. The enhancement pattern seen with MR is identical to the pattern on CT.

Management

In cases where characteristic findings are absent or atypical features are present it may be difficult to differentiate intrahepatic cholangiocarcinoma from other primary or secondary liver lesions. In such cases, the use of fine needle aspiration may be warranted for definitive characterization.

Further Reading

1. Soyer P, Bluemke DA, Reichle R. et al. Imaging of Intrahepatic Cholangiocarcinoma: Peripheral Cholangiocarcinoma. *Am J Roentgenol.* 1995; *165*: 1427–1431.

History

▶ Previously healthy 65-year-old woman with chronic right upper abdominal pain.

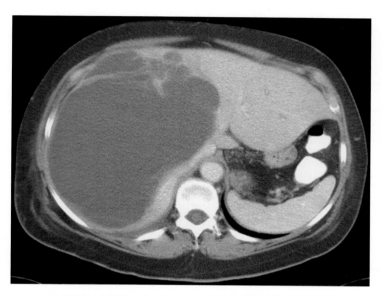

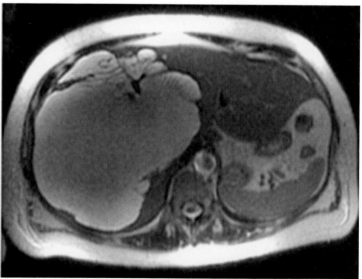

Case 99 Biliary Cystadenoma

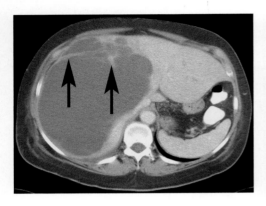 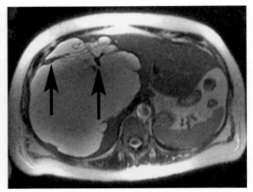

Findings

CT (left image) obtained during the portal venous phase shows a large solitary cystic mass replacing most of the right lobe of liver. Thick nodular septations (black arrows) are present in portions of the mass. T2-weighted single-shot MR (right image) shows the mass to be cystic and shows the septations (arrows) more prominently.

Differential Diagnosis

► Echinococcal cyst: usually does not have enhancement of septations and intracystic components. Serology may help to establish the diagnosis.
► Resolving intrahepatic hemorrhage: requires history of trauma.
► Simple hepatic cyst: should not have thick nodular septations.
► Biliary cystadenocarcinoma: uncommon and difficult to distinguish with certainty from biliary cystadenoma unless metastases are present.

Teaching Points

Biliary cystadenomas are uncommon and typically present in middle-aged to elderly women as a large solitary benign or low-grade malignant cystic liver mass that may have thickened septations or nodularity at cross-sectional imaging. Vague increasing symptoms of abdominal discomfort or pain may lead patients to seek medical attention. Frank malignancy is uncommon, but may occasionally occur. While these lesions are believed to arise from the bile duct wall, upstream bile duct dilatation is not typically an associated finding. At resection, histopathology reveals ovarian-like stroma of the cyst wall and septations. Primary cystic liver malignancies are distinctly rare and should be low on the differential diagnosis for the de novo finding of biliary cystic lesions. Biliary cystadenomas are believed by some to be pre-malignant, and malignant biliary cystadenocarcinomas may be indistinguishable from the more common benign cystadenoma.

Management

Since these lesions may progress in size and carry a low likelihood of being frankly malignant, curative surgical resection is the most accepted treatment.

Further Reading

1. Anderson SW, Kruskal JB, Kane RA. Benign hepatic tumors and iatrogenic pseudotumors *RadioGraphics*. 2009;29(1):211–229.

History

► Previously healthy 43-year-old woman with no risk factors for cirrhosis presents with acute upper abdominal pain and decreased hematocrit.

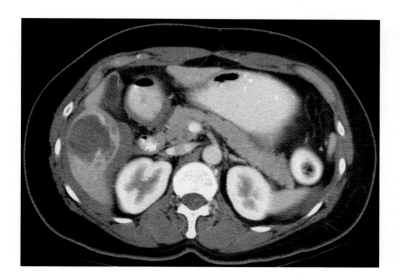

Case 100 Hepatic Angiosarcoma

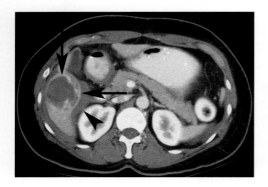

Findings

CT obtained during the portal venous phase shows a heterogeneous mass (arrows) in the liver tip with areas of hyperenhancement and areas of poor enhancement. Dense fluid (arrowhead) surrounds the liver tip, consistent with intraperitoneal hemorrhage.

Differential Diagnosis

▶ Hepatocellular carcinoma: may present as a solitary mass with hemorrhagic rupture. More commonly occurs in patients with chronic liver disease and cirrhosis.

▶ Hepatic adenoma: occurs predominantly in young women on oral contraceptives and patients with glycogen storage disease. These tumors may undergo spontaneous life-threatening hemorrhage.

▶ Hypervascular liver metastasis: patients usually have a history of a known malignancy.

Teaching Points

Hepatic angiosarcomas are rare tumors that have a highly variable appearance at presentation. They may have components that are hyper- and hypovascular, may have a pseudocapsule, may be large at the time of discovery, may hemorrhage or rupture, and may show derangement of associated vessels. Unfortunately these findings are nonspecific, so these tumors are difficult to diagnose without tissue sampling or resection. Risk factors for angiosarcoma include exposure to vinyl chloride, arsenic, or prior administration of thorotrast, which is a now discontinued intravenous hepatosplenic contrast material. Though hepatic angiosarcomas are the most common primary hepatic mesenchymal malignancy, other non-hepatocellular carcinoma malignancies to consider include epithelioid hemangioendothelioma, liposarcoma, undifferentiated embryonal sarcoma, leiomyosarcoma, and malignant fibrous histiocytoma.

Management

The prognosis for primary liver sarcomas, including hepatic angiosarcoma, remains poor. The mainstays of treatment are complete surgical resection and adjuvant chemotherapy. Recognition of the absence of risk factors for hepatocellular carcinoma may raise the preoperative concern for a liver sarcoma.

Further Readings

1. Yu RS, Chen Y, Jiang B, Wang LH, Xu XF. Primary hepatic sarcomas: CT findings. *Eur Radiol.* 2008 Oct;*18*(10):2196–2205.
2. Almogy G, Lieberman S, Gips M, Pappo O, Edden Y, Jurim O, Simon Slasky B, Uzieli B, Eid A. Clinical outcomes of surgical resections for primary liver sarcoma in adults: results from a single centre. *Eur J Surg Oncol.* 2004 May;*30*(4):421–427.

History

▸ 73-year-old female patient with left-sided back pain.

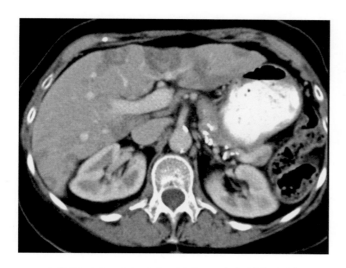

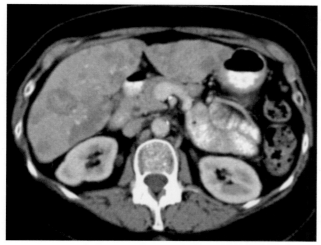

Case 101 Epithelioid Hemangioendothelioma

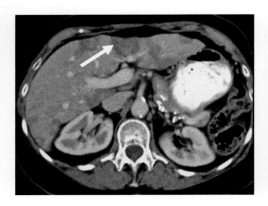 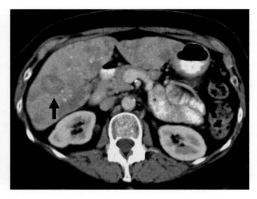

Findings

CT images show innumerable hypoenhancing lesions that are scattered throughout the liver parenchyma. The lesions have a predominant peripheral location and coalescence in some areas. Several of the lesions are associated with capsular retraction (white arrow). All lesions have central enhancement (black arrow).

Differential Diagnosis

► Hepatic metastases: may cause capsular retraction and demonstrate central enhancement. Diffuse liver metastases often are associated with a known primary neoplasm. Capsular contracture associated with liver metastasis usually occurs following treatment.

► Intrahepatic cholangiocarcinoma: commonly causes capsular retraction and shows delayed central enhancement. Usually intrahepatic cholangiocarcinoma is associated with peripheral biliary duct obstruction and the multifocality would be uncommon.

Teaching Points

Hepatic epithelioid hemagioendothelioma is a rare liver tumor of vascular origin. At present, no risk factors or specific causes have been identified. Hepatic epithelioid hemagioendothelioma is found typically in young adults, mostly middle-aged women, with common age range of 18 to 48 years. Although the tumor is considered malignant, it carries a better prognosis than other primary hepatic malignancies, even in the presence of distant metastases. Relatively specific imaging findings of hepatic epithelioid hemagioendothelioma that have been reported previously include the presence of multilayered concentric target-shaped nodules that are mostly located in the periphery of the liver; associated capsular retraction; and presence of the "lollipop" sign, which is characterized by a thrombosed vessel ending at the periphery of the tumor nodule. Occasionally this entity may present as a solitary liver lesion.

Management

The clinical course of hepatic epithelioid hemagioendothelioma is variable and unpredictable. Twenty percent of patients die within two years after presentation; another 20 percent have an extended survival of 5 to 28 years, regardless of whether they undergo treatment.

Further Reading

1. Earnest F, Johnson CD. Hepatic epithelioid hemangioendothelioma. *Radiology.* 2006; *240*: 295–298.

History

► 58-year-old man with abdominal pain, right hip and thigh pain, and weight loss.

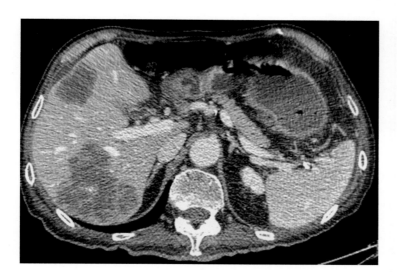

Case 102 Metastasis to the Liver

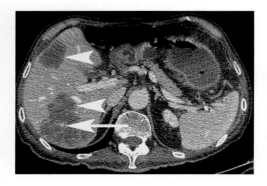

Findings

CT shows two lobulated low-attenuation masses (arrowheads) in the liver (short arrow) with heterogeneous enhancement. The more posterior mass shows a focus of hyperattenuation within the mass, consistent with calcification. This patient had a known mucinous colonic adenocarcinoma.

Differential Diagnosis

▶ Lymphoma: often associated with lymphadenopathy.
▶ Hepatic abscesses: may be fungal, pyogenic (bacterial), or mycobacterial, and are usually associated with signs of systemic infection. Fungal abscesses are usually small and multiple. Pyogenic abscesses may initially "cluster" together, prior to coalescing.
▶ Hepatic cysts: non-enhancing, fluid-attenuation masses with sharp, well defined borders.

Teaching Points

The liver is the most common site of metastases for gastrointestinal primary malignancies, and is commonly involved by a wide range of other malignancies, including lung and breast cancer and melanoma. Liver metastases may be hypovascular or hypervascular and have a variable appearance on CT. Most adenocarcinoma metastases are hypoattenuating compared to liver parenchyma on portal venous phase CT. Arterial phase imaging is helpful in primary carcinomas known to have hypervascular metastases (i.e, neuroendocrine tumors, carcinoid, renal cell carcinoma, melanoma, thyroid cancer). FDG PET, with or without associated combined CT, has shown increased sensitivity in detecting hepatic metastases when compared with CT alone. Calcified hepatic metastases, though uncommon, are most often seen with mucinous colonic adenocarcinoma.

Management

Particularly with gastrointestinal primaries, improved survival may be obtained with systemic therapy supplemented by surgical resection or ablation of liver metastases when the metastases are few in number. Therefore, the location, number, and size of liver metastases are important to describe in radiological reports.

Further Readings

1. Kinkel K, Lu Y, Both M. Detection of hepatic metastases from cancers of the gastrointestinal tract by using noninvasive imaging methods (US, CT, MR imaging, PET): a meta-analysis. *Radiology*. Sep 2002; *224*(3): 748–756.
2. Stoupis C, Taylor HM, Paley MR, Buetow PC, Marre S, Baer HU, Vock P, Ros PR. The Rocky liver: radiologic-pathologic correlation of calcified hepatic masses. *RadioGraphics*. May 1998; *18*:675–685.

History

▶ 65-year-old man status post orthotopic liver transplantation 5 days prior.

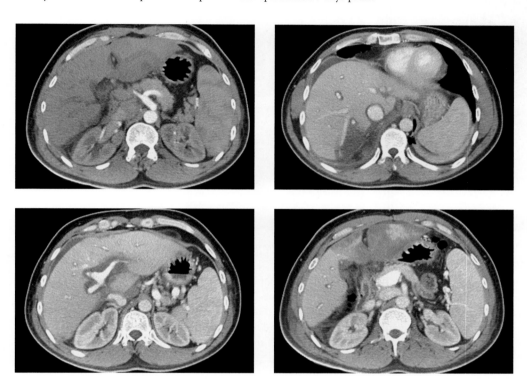

Case 103 Post-Liver Transplant Ischemia

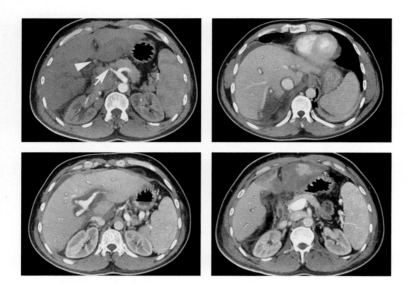

Findings

Intravenous contrast-enhanced CT in the arterial phase (upper left image) shows abrupt occlusion of the hepatic artery (arrow) and high attenuation thrombus in the distal hepatic artery in the liver hilum (arrowhead). The early portal venous phase images show patent portal veins, lack of intrahepatic arterial opacification, periportal low attenuation edema and multiple, wedge- and geographic-shaped areas of peripheral low attenuation in both lobes. There is a small amount of perihepatic fluid.

Differential Diagnosis

► Hepatic trauma: may also result in hepatic infarction if there is arterial injury. Other findings of traumatic injury such as laceration, intraparenchymal hemorrhage, subcapsular hematoma, and peritoneal hemorrhage may be present.

► Focal hepatic steatosis: may mimic infarction when located in the subcapsular regions. It is typically geographic- or wedge-shaped. There is normal opacification of the hepatic vasculature.

Teaching Points

Hepatic artery thrombosis is a feared complication of liver transplantation. Hepatic transplant ischemia and infarction is due to hepatic artery pathology 85 percent of the time, and less commonly due to portal vein thrombosis. Infarcted regions of the liver may become necrotic and liquefy. Superinfection may also occur. Extensive infarction leads to graft failure. Bile duct ischemia may complicate hepatic artery thrombosis because the hepatic artery is the sole blood supply to the bile ducts. Ischemic bile ducts may manifest as dilatation, strictures, leaks, or all of these findings.

Management

Balloon angioplasty or thrombectomy may be used to open the thrombosed artery. If unsuccessful, retransplantation may be required.

Further Readings

1. Segel MC, Zajko AB, Bowen A, et al. Hepatic artery thrombosis after liver transplantation: radiologic evaluation. *Am J Roentgenol.* 1986;*146*(1):137–141.
2. Quiroga S, Sebastia MC, Margarit C, Castells L, Boye R, Alvarez-Castells A. Complications of orthotopic liver transplantation: spectrum of findings with helical CT. *RadioGraphics.* 2001;*21*(5):1085–1102.

History

► 43-year-old man found unconscious in the street.

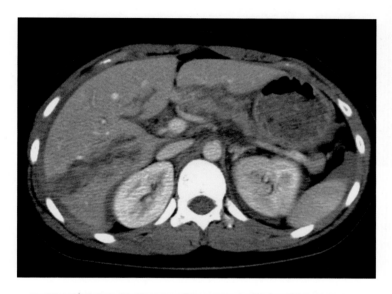

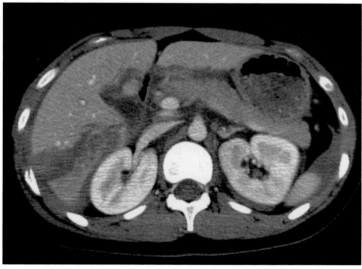

Case 104 Traumatic Hepatic and Pancreatic Laceration with Hemoperitoneum

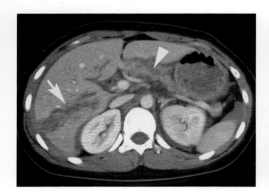 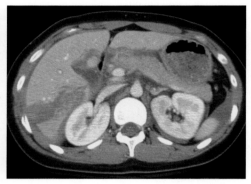

Findings

Intravenous contrast-enhanced CT images show linear areas of low attenuation in the right lobe of the liver and pancreas (arrowhead), compatible with hepatic and pancreatic laceration. The hepatic laceration extends through the hepatic capsule and there is high-attenuation ascites, which is consistent with hemoperitoneum.

Differential Diagnosis

▶ Spontaneous hepatic rupture and hemorrhage: may occur in patients with: tumors such as hepatocellular adenoma, hepatocellular carcinoma, metastasis, and angiosarcoma; coagulopathies; collagen vascular disease; peliosis; and in pregnant women with eclampsia or preeclampsia. Hemorrhagic hepatic tumors typically have a rounded configuration, but may be difficult to distinguish from focal intraparenchymal hemorrhage from other causes.

▶ Traumatic hepatic contusion: ill-defined areas of hypoattenuation that may be admixed with high-attenuation hemorrhage.

Teaching Points

Hepatic laceration may occur from compressive or shearing forces on the liver. The posterior right lobe of the liver is the most common location of injury because of its large size and proximity to the spine and ribs. While lacerations are the most common liver injury to blunt force trauma, the spectrum of injuries also includes subcapsular and intraparenchymal hematomas and injuries to the hepatic vasculature. Lacerations are characteristically linear, branching low attenuation regions with the liver. It is important to assess the proximity of the laceration to critical vessels such as the inferior vena cava, portal veins, and hepatic veins as well as involvement of the bile ducts or capsule and the presence or absence of active hemorrhage.

Management

Unstable patients or patients with active hemorrhage are managed surgically. Embolization may also be performed with active hemorrhage. Patients that are hemodynamically stable may be managed nonsurgically. If a patient has persistent or worsening symptoms, a repeat CT should be performed. Follow-up CT in stable patients is controversial.

Further Reading

1. Yoon W, Jeong YY, Kim JK, et al. CT in blunt liver trauma. *RadioGraphics*. 2005;25(1):87–104.

History:

▶ 48-year-old man with hepatitis C cirrhosis presents with elevated alpha feto protein (AFP). MRI obtained to evaluate for hepatocellular carcinoma.

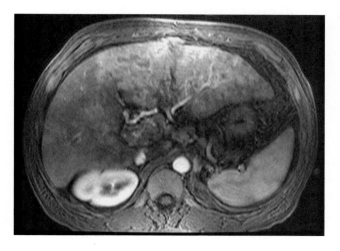

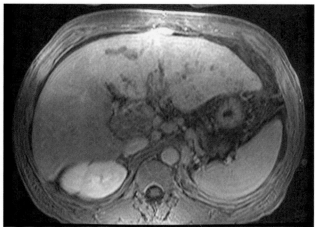

Case 105   Hepatic Cirrhosis with Portal Vein Tumor Thrombus

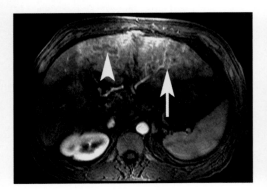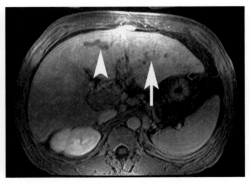

Findings

T1 post-gadolinium arterial (left) and late portal venous phase images (right) show heterogeneous left hepatic lobe hyperenhancement. Left lateral portal vein expansion, arterial phase hyperenhancement, and venous phase washout (arrow) is consistent with tumor thrombus. Left medial lobe portal vein also shows tumor thrombus (arrowhead).

Differential Diagnosis

▶ Bland portal vein thrombus: the portal vein should not enhance during any phase of imaging. Associated heterogeneous liver parenchyma hyperenhancement may occur.
▶ Portal vein pylephlebitis: portal vein mural thickening and mural hyperenhancement with portal vein thrombus in the setting of sepsis.

Teaching Points

Portal vein tumor thrombus from hepatocellular carcinoma must be considered whenever heterogeneous liver enhancement is seen in a cirrhotic liver or in a patient at risk for hepatocellular carcinoma. Obstruction of normal portal venous inflow results in increased arterial flow into the affected liver segments and frequently results in arterial phase parenchymal hyperenhancement. Nonvisualization of a normal portal vein at imaging should prompt a search for a tumor that either obliterates the portal vein or that expands and distorts to the point that the portal vein is difficult to recognize. Delayed imaging may show contrast material washout from the portal vein rather than enhancement similar to the blood pool. Discrete hepatocellular carcinomas must be sought, though the tumor may be obscured by the heterogeneous liver enhancement caused by portal vein obstruction. In contrast, bland thrombus of the portal vein typically does not cause substantial expansion of the vein, nor should enhancing tissue be seen in the portal vein.

Management

Portal vein tumor thrombus generally precludes curative liver transplantation for patients with hepatocellular carcinoma. Multiphase imaging or dedicated US may be obtained to confirm the presence of tumor thrombus.

Further Reading

1. Lee HK, Park SJ, Yi BH, Yeon EK, Kim JH, Hong HS. Portal vein thrombosis: CT features. *Abdom Imaging*. 2008; 33:72–79.

History

▶ 69-year-old man with history of non-Hodgkin's lymphoma and autologous bone marrow transplant.

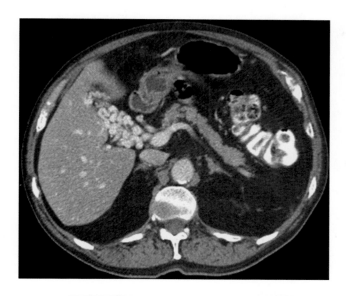

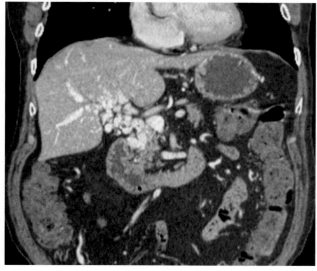

Case 106 Cavernous Transformation of the Portal Vein

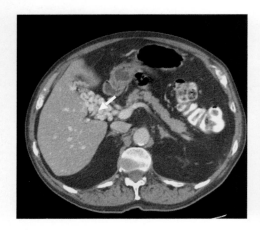 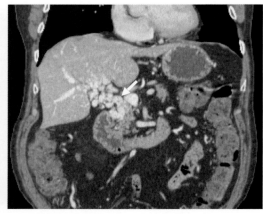

Findings

CT images obtained during the portal venous phase shows serpigenous enhancing veins (arrow) in the porta hepatis. The main portal vein is not visualized.

Differential Diagnosis

► Tumor thrombus in the portal vein: may expand the portal vein and enhance. Tumor thrombus occurs when there is a malignant liver mass such as hepatocellular carcinoma or cholangiocarcinoma.
► Hepatoduodenal ligament lymph nodes or mass: usually less serpentine in shape and less enhancement.

Teaching Points

Cavernous transformation of the portal vein occurs as a consequence of extrahepatic portal vein thrombosis and occlusion. Numerous tortuous venous collaterals develop over a variable time course, ranging from a week to a year. Collateral veins develop from biliary, gastric, pericholecystic veins, the partially recanalized portal vein, and portosystemic collateral channels that drain variably into the left and right portal veins and the vasa vasorum. The collaterals may extend into the liver. On CT, numerous, serpiginous veins are seen in the expected region of the portal vein. They enhance during the portal venous phase. On ultrasound, flow within collateral veins is generally hepatopetal, low velocity, and fairly monophasic, lacking the slight pulsatility seen in the normal portal vein flow. Portal venous thrombosis can be associated with hepatic parenchymal perfusion abnormalities from a compensatory increase in arterial inflow or occasionally bile duct obstruction due to mass effect by the collateral veins on the common duct. Atrophy of the left lateral segment and hypertrophy of the left medial segment and the caudate lobe may also occur in these cases. Causes of portal vein thrombosis include reduced portal flow from underlying hepatic parenchymal disease, abdominal sepsis (infectious, abdominal inflammation), and hypercoagulable states.

Management

Ninety percent of patients with cavernous transformation of the portal vein have portal hypertension. Variceal hemorrhage and splenomegaly are management challenges because TIPS (transjugular intrahepatic portosystemic shunt) is not a feasible option for management.

Further Reading

1. Vilgrain V, Condat B, Bureau C, et al. Atrophy-Hypertrophy Complex in Patients with Cavernous Transformation of the Portal Vein: CT evaluation. *Radiology.* 2006; *241*(1):149–155.

History

▶ 22-year-old man with fever, malaise, and abdominal pain.

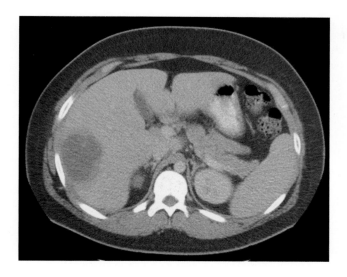

Case 107 Pyogenic Abscess

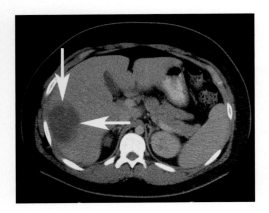

Findings

CT image of the upper abdomen show a low attenuation cystic lesion in the right hepatic lobe (arrows).

Differential Diagnosis

► Amebic Abscess: has very similar imaging characteristics to a pyogenic abscess.
► Treated metastatic disease: patient history of prior neoplasm and lack of fever, leukocytosis are clues to the correct diagnosis.
► Biliary cystadenocarcinoma: encapsulated complex cystic lesion occurring most commonly in middle-aged women.
► Hepatic hydatid cyst: Cystic liver mass that may have varied appearances, including peripheral daughter cysts. Will occasionally show curvilinear or peri-cyst calcification.

Teaching Points

Pyogenic liver abscess is a localized collection of pus in the liver, typically from a polymicrobial bacterial infection. Pyogenic abscess accounts for 80 percent of liver abscesses, with amebic abscess (from *Entamoeba histolytica*) being responsible for another 10 percent, and fungal abscess (typically *Candida*) comprising the remaining 10 percent. Causes of pyogenic abscess are multifactorial. Biliary disease with ascending cholangitis and portal vein pylephlebitis from diverticulitis, appendicitis, or inflammatory bowel disease account for the majority of cases in the Western world. Other causes included hepatic arterial septicemia, triggered perhaps by endocarditis or osteomyelitis, direct extension from perforated duodenal ulcer, or subphrenic abscess or from blunt or penetrating trauma. Patients present most commonly with right upper quadrant pain, malaise, and fever. If the infection spreads to the subphrenic region, right lower lobe atelectasis or a right pleural effusion may be present. The diagnostic study of choice is contrast-enhanced CT of the abdomen and pelvis, which will show a rim-enhancing fluid collection in the liver.

Management

Antibiotics and percutaneous abscess drainage with catheter placement is the procedure of choice for treatment of pyogenic liver abscess, with success rates of greater than 90 percent. For smaller abscesses, treatment with needle aspiration with antibiotics has also been shown to be effective.

Further Reading

1. Kurland, JE, Brann OS. Pyogenic and amebic liver abscesses. *Curr Gastroenterology Rep.* 2004:6: 273–279.

History

▸ 38-year-old man with fever and abdominal pain.

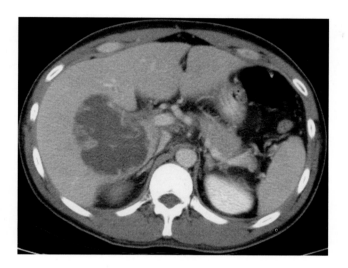

Case 108 Amebic Abscess

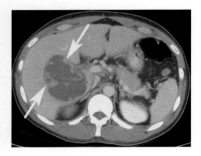

Findings

CT image through the upper abdomen shows a cystic mass with mural irregularity (arrows) in the right posterior liver.

Differential Diagnosis

► Cystic/necrotic post-treatment metastatic disease: can look very similar to amebic abscess. History of primary malignancy and correlation with prior studies is usually diagnostic.
► Biliary cystadenocarcinoma: rare rim-enhancing cystic mass in the liver that may have thick mural septations or nodules, typically occurring in middle-aged women. Unlike amebic abscess, these typically lack any surrounding inflammatory change and are not associated with sepsis.
► Pyogenic abscess: indistinguishable from amebic abscess by imaging characteristics.
► Hydatid cyst: large well defined cystic liver mass. The appearance of multiple smaller peripheral daughter cysts and/or rim calcification is suggestive. Subacute onset of symptoms and history of travel to an area where the disease is endemic are useful discriminators.

Teaching Points

Amebic liver abscess is the most frequent extra-intestinal manifestation of *Entamoeba histolytica* infection. Approximately 10 percent of the world population is infected by contaminated drinking water, the vast majority in developing countries in Central America, India, and Southeast Asia. Patients typically present with acute to subacute symptoms of right upper quadrant pain, tender hepatomegaly, and diarrhea with mucus. History of recent travel to a region where the disease is endemic is critical in narrowing the differential diagnosis. Contrast-enhanced CT shows a sensitivity of 88 to 95 percent for identifying amebic liver abscesses. Typical finding is a rim-enhancing fluid collection in the liver. Amebic abscesses are more common in the right hepatic lobe (72 percent), presumably due to the right lobe receiving the majority of its blood supply from the superior mesenteric vein. Potential complications include rupture through the diaphragm into the chest with pulmonary abscess and hydropneumothorax, or intraperitoneal rupture with amebic peritonitis.

Management

Most uncomplicated amebic abscesses can be treated successfully with amebicidal drug therapy alone. An oral course of metronidazole for 10 days has been shown to be curative in 90 percent of uncomplicated cases, with resolution of symptoms within three days in most patients. Percutaneous drainage is reserved for cases in which there is a high risk of abscess rupture, such as abscesses 5 cm or larger in size, failure to observe a clinical response to amebicidal treatment, or if the collection cannot be reliably differentiated from a pyogenic abscess.

Further Readings

1. Sharma MP, Ahuja V. Management of amebic and pyogenic liver abscesses. *Indian J of Gastroenterology* 2001:*20*:C33–C36.
2. Hughes MA, Petri WA Jr. Amebic Liver Abscess. *Inf Dis Clin North Am*. 2000:*14*(3):565–582.
3. Rajak CL, Gupta S, Jain S, Chawla Y, Gulati M, Suri S. Percutaneous treatment of liver abscesses: needle aspiration versus catheter drainage. *Am J Roentgenol*. 1998:*170*(4):1035–1039.

History

▶ 23-year-old female patient with low-grade fever and abdominal pain.

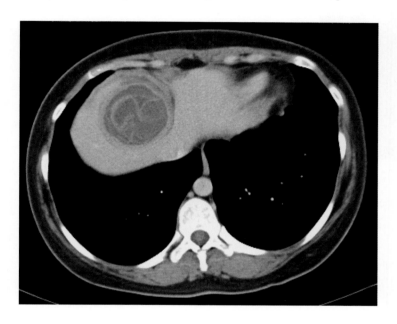

Case 109 Hepatic Echinococcal (Hydatid) Cyst

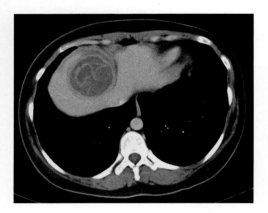

Findings

CT shows a solitary complex hepatic cyst. The cyst has a thick enhancing wall and contains a delaminated internal wall ("water lily" sign).

Differential Diagnosis

► Pyogenic abscess: often multilocular and hypoattenuating on CT, with an irregular enhancing contour and surrounding edema. The presence of gas, although rare, can be diagnostically helpful.
► Amebic abscess: similar appearance to pyogenic abscess. Patients are often acutely and severely ill with fever and abdominal pain upon presentation.
► E. multilocularis: a rare form of echinococcal infection. Multilocular hypoattenuating appearance on CT, with cysts measuring less than 1 cm in size. Minimal enhancement and central liquefaction is common, and these lesions often mimic pyogenic infections.

Teaching Points

There are two forms of echinococcus infection, *E. granulosus and E. multilocularis.* Hydatid (*E. granulosus*) disease is the more common parasitic disease and is endemic to the Mediterranean basin and other sheep-raising areas. Hydatid cysts are composed of three histopathologic layers: the outer pericyst, the inner endocyst, and the interleaved ectocyst. Biochemical analysis usually reveals eosinophilia; however, serologic testing is positive in only 25 percent of patients. Cyst maturation is characterized by peripheral daughter cyst development. On ultrasound, the imaging appearance is variable, ranging from cystic to solid appearing pseudotumors. Daughter cysts, peripheral calcification, and delaminated endocysts (water lily sign) may be present. Potential complications of hydatid disease include cyst rupture, diaphragmatic and abdominal wall involvement, peritoneal seeding, portal vein involvement, biliary communication, and hematogenous spread.

Management

Although previously not recommended, following medical pretreatment with mebendazole, percutaneous drainage, and cyst sclerosis is now widely accepted. Complications, including superinfection of the treated cyst cavity and biliary communication, are possible.

Further Reading

1. Mortele KJ, Segatto E, Ros PR, et al. The Infected Liver: Radiologic-Pathologic Correlation *RadioGraphics.* 2004; *24*: 937–955.

History

▶ 48-year-old man with lethargy and increasing abdominal girth. Laboratory studies reveal a moderate increase in the serum alkaline phosphatase and elevated angiotensin converting enzyme levels.

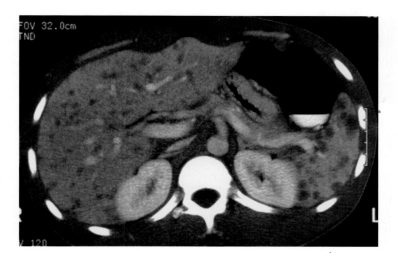

Case 110 Hepatic and Splenic Sarcoidosis

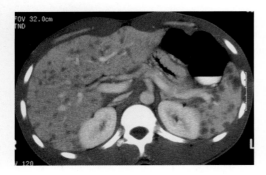

Findings

Intravenous contrast-enhanced CT shows numerous hypoattenuating small masses in the liver and spleen.

Differential Diagnosis

▶ Metastatic disease: demonstrates a wide spectrum of appearance on imaging studies and is indistinguishable from hepatic sarcoid. Splenic metastasis is uncommon.

▶ Lymphoma: may present similarly with multiple small lesions in the liver and spleen.

▶ Microabscesses: may have a similar appearance with small focal low-attenuation lesions scattered throughout the liver, especially in immunocompromised patients.

Teaching Points

Sarcoidosis is a systemic granulomatous disease. The liver is reportedly involved in up to 79 percent of patients with the disease at histopathology, but clinically significant liver disease is present in 5 percent of patients. The spectrum of disease in the liver varies from asymptomatic elevations in liver enzymes to end-stage chronic liver disease. CT may show hepatomegaly, parenchymal heterogeneity, multifocal nodules in the liver, or confluent lymphadenopathy, and occasionally, small hypoattenuating or large confluent nodules. Upper abdominal lymphadenopathy may be present. In the most severe disease, cirrhosis occurs. Biopsy of the liver reveals noncaseating granulomas in the portal and periportal regions of the hepatic lobules.

Management

The treatment of hepatic sarcoid varies with disease severity. Corticosteroids have been used as first-line treatment. Other immunosuppressives, including methotrexate, are alternative agents. Organ transplantation may be considered for advanced sarcoidosis.

Further Readings

1. Warshauer D, Dumbleton S, Molina P, et al. Abdominal CT findings in sarcoidosis: radiologic and clinical correlation. *Radiology*. 1994 Jul; *192*(1): 93–98.
2. Harder H, Büchler M, Fröhlich B, et al. Extrapulmonary sarcoidosis of liver and pancreas: A case report and review of literature. *World J Gastroenterol* . 2007 May 7; *13*(17): 2504–2509.
3. Britt A, Francis I, Glazer G, et al. Sarcoidosis: abdominal manifestations at CT. *Radiology*. 1991 Jan; *178*(1): 91–94.

History

▶ 30-year-old female with leukemia and status post-liver transplant.

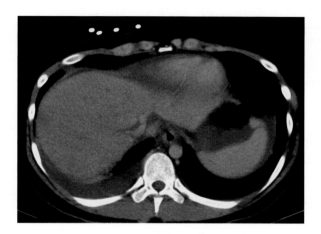

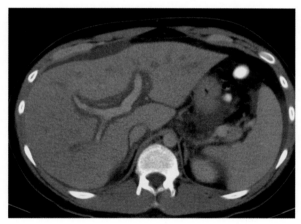

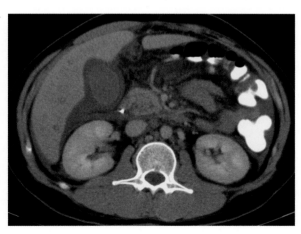

Case 111 Veno-Occlusive Disease (VOD)

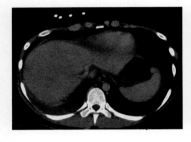 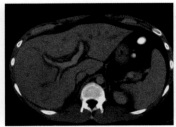 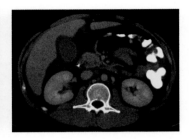

Findings

CT shows hepatomegaly and perihepatic ascites. Attenuated hepatic veins, hepatic heterogeneity, periportal edema, and gallbladder wall edema are present. Findings of VOD were confirmed with transjugular liver biopsy.

Differential Diagnosis

▶ Budd-Chiari syndrome: occluded hepatic veins or IVC with intrahepatic venous collaterals. The caudate lobe and central liver segments are spared due to differential drainage of these segments through the caudate vein.
▶ Passive hepatic congestion: hepatomegaly, heterogeneous parenchyma, periportal edema, gallbladder wall thickening, and perihepatic ascites in the setting of right-sized heart failure. Hepatic veins and IVC are dilated and show reflux of contrast from the heart.

Teaching Points

VOD is a progressive inflammatory process that occurs at the level of the post-sinusoidal hepatic veins leading to non-thrombotic venous occlusion. It is most frequently seen after stem-cell transplant or solid organ transplant with an incidence approaching 70 percent. High dose chemotherapy causes endothelial injury leading to thrombus formation. It usually occurs 10 to 20 days after a regimen containing cyclophosphamide, but can occur up to nine weeks after. Other associations include alcoholic liver disease, use of oral contraceptives, toxic oil ingestion, use of terbinafine, prior radiation, ingestion of herbal teas or travel to Jamaica ("bush tea" disease). It presents as a clinical syndrome of ascites, hepatomegaly, abdominal pain, and jaundice secondary to hyperbilirubinemia. On US there is hepatomegaly, ascites, and attenuated hepatic veins. Decreased or reversed flow in the segmental or main portal veins and increased resistive index in the hepatic artery may be present. MRI shows hepatomegaly, ascites, heterogeneous hypointense signal intensity of the hepatic parenchyma on T1-WI, and heterogeneous hyperintense signal intensity on T2-WI consistent with hepatic congestion. There is associated periportal edema, gallbladder wall thickening, and increased signal in the gallbladder wall on T2. Patchy enhancement of the hepatic parenchyma occurs with multiple enhancing "dots" that represent intrahepatic venous collaterals.

Management

VOD can be prevented by using non-myeloablative chemotherapy regimens and by using prophylaxis with ursodeoxycholic acid or defibriotide. Treatment is usually supportive and spontaneous recovery occurs in 70 to 85 percent of cases.

Further Reading

1. Mortele KM, Vlierberghe H, Wiesner W, et al. Hepatic veno-occlusive disease: MRI findings. *Abdom Imaging*. 2002; *27*:523–526.

Part 8   **Gallbladder**

History

▶ 66-year-old woman with right upper quadrant pain.

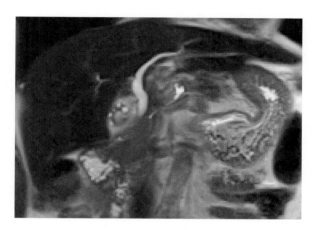

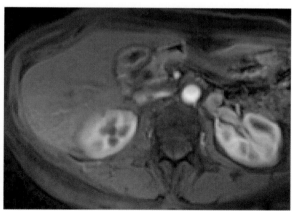

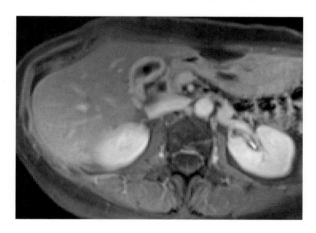

Case 112   Adenomyomatosis Hyperplasia

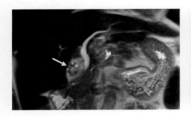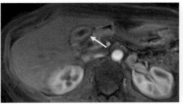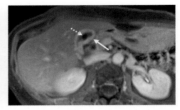

Findings

T2-weighted MR image (left) shows a thickened gallbladder wall with multiple small intramural T2 hyperintense foci (arrow). Enhanced T1-weighted image (middle) shows diffuse early mucosal enhancement (arrow). Delayed enhanced T1-weighted image (right) shows diffuse mural enhancement (arrow) and a gallstone in the gallbladder lumen (arrowhead).

Differential Diagnosis

▶ Gallbladder carcinoma: can appear as a focal or diffuse gallbladder wall thickening. The wall thickening tends to be irregular, eccentric, or asymmetric and lacks normal mucosal enhancement. Finding associated features such as lymphadenopathy, invasion into the liver, and evidence of hematogenous metastases is helpful to suggest the diagnosis.

▶ Inflammatory and noninflammatory wall thickening: cholecystitis, heart failure, cirrhosis, hepatitis, renal failure, portal hypertension and AIDS cholangiopathy may be distinguished by the clinical setting and associated imaging features.

Teaching Points

Adenomyomatous hyperplasia (also called adenomyomatosis) of the gallbladder frequently coexists with cholelithiasis, but no causative relationship has been proven. It is more frequently seen in women and occasionally manifests with persistent right upper quadrant pain. Pathologically, it is characterized by mucosal hyperplasia and thickening of the muscular layer of the gallbladder. Mucosal herniations into the muscular layer are called Rokitansky-Aschoff sinuses, which when filled with bile can appear as high T2 signal foci in the gallbladder wall. This appearance is referred to as the "pearl necklace" sign. The "rosary" sign is the CT finding of enhancing epithelium within intramural diverticula surrounded by the hypoattenuating hypertrophied muscular layer. These signs are highly specific in distinguishing adenomyomatosis from gallbladder cancer. Adenomyomatosis may manifest as diffuse wall thickening, focal segmental annular thickening or a localized mass which is usually at the fundus and has a sessile or semilunar shape. On contrast-enhanced CT and MRI images, the diffuse type demonstrates early mucosal enhancement with subsequent transmural enhancement.

Management

Adenomyomatosis requires no follow-up or biopsy. In cases where it is difficult to distinguish adenomyomatosis from gallbladder malignancy, short-term imaging follow-up or cholecystectomy should be considered.

Further Reading

1. Ching BH, Yeh BM, Westphalen AC, Joe BN, Qayyum A, Coakley FV. CT differentiation of adenomyomatosis and gallbladder cancer. *Am J Roentgenol.* 2007 Jul;*189*(1):62–66.

History

▶ 80-year-old woman with elevated liver function tests and right upper quadrant pain.

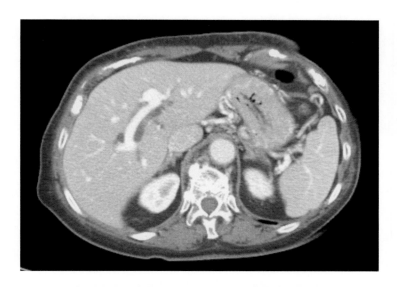

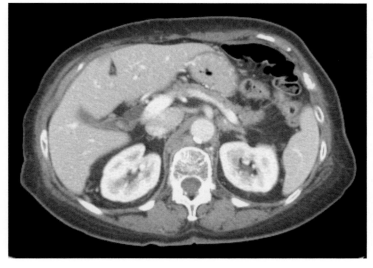

Case 113 Mirizzi Syndrome

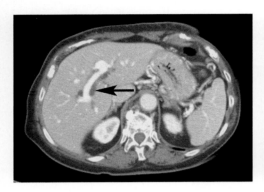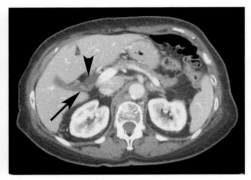

Findings

CT shows dilated intrahepatic bile duct (arrow left image) and an impacted stone in the cystic duct (arrow right image) adjacent to the dilated common duct (arrowhead).

Differential Diagnosis

► Choledocholithiasis: will typically appear as an intraluminal filling defect within the common duct rather than in the cystic duct.
► Acute cholecystitis/gallbladder carcinoma: Acute inflammation with focal enlargement of the gallbladder or a gallbladder mass may cause mass effect on and dilate the common duct and can simulate Mirizzi syndrome.

Teaching Points

Mirizzi syndrome is a rare cause of obstructive jaundice, occurring in less than 0.5 percent of all patients treated for gallstone disease. The pathogenesis involves a long common sheath enveloping the cystic duct and common hepatic duct. A gallstone that lodges in the cystic duct will then cause mass effect on the common hepatic duct and thereby obstruct the biliary tract. Mirizzi syndrome may result in erosion by the stone through the cystic duct to cause a cholecystobiliary fistula. There are no consistent or unique clinical features to distinguish Mirizzi syndrome from other forms of obstructive jaundice. Careful ultrasound imaging can demonstrate the presence of a large impacted cystic duct stone with intrahepatic biliary dilation, and an abrupt change in caliber of the biliary duct at the site of cystic duct insertion should raise concern for Mirizzi syndrome. CT and ultrasound have a similar sensitivity of 23 to 46 percent, but CT is superior in identifying other obstructive causes such as gallbladder cancer, cholangiocarcinoma, or metastatic tumor. Direct cholangiography, ERCP, or MRCP can assist in defining the precise ductal anatomy and the presence or absence of stricture or fistula to guide surgery.

Management

For relatively uncomplicated cases, a conventional cholecystectomy with common duct exploration and T-tube placement is recommended. In cases with a cholecystobiliary fistula, a choledochoplasty or biliary-enteric anastomosis may be needed.

Further Reading

1. Johnson LW, Sehon JK, Lee WC, Zibari GB, McDonald JC. Mirizzi's syndrome: experience from a multi-institutional review. *Am Surg.* 2001 Jan;67(1):11–14.

History

▶ 72-year-old woman presenting with abdominal pain and distention, nausea, and vomiting.

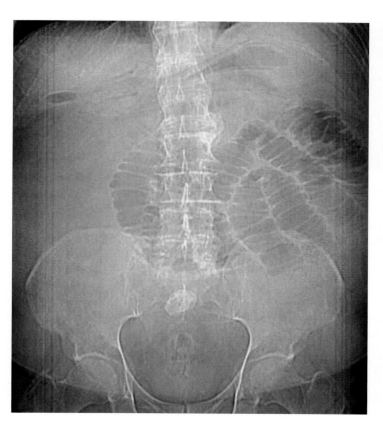

Case 114   Gallstone Ileus

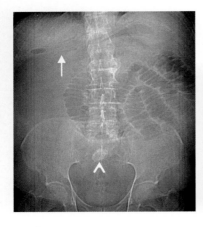
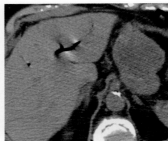
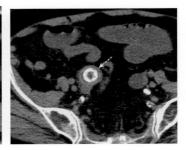

Findings

Supine abdominal radiograph (left) image shows pneumobilia (white arrow). Dilated small bowel and a radiopaque gallstone (arrowhead) projecting over the pelvis suggest a mechanical obstruction. CT shows the pneumobilia (center) and more inferiorly (right) the gallstone (dashed arrow) impacted in the distal jejunum, which was the transition point for the small bowel obstruction. The distal segments of small bowel are decompressed.

Differential Diagnosis

▶ Intussusception: transition point usually shows a target appearance at cross-section that corresponds to outer layer of segment of bowel (intussuscepiens) within inner layer of distal small bowel (intussusceptum). No pneumobilia or gallstone is present.

▶ Dropped gallstone: stones dropped during laparoscopic cholecystectomy are usually within the peritoneal cavity. No evidence of bowel obstruction or transition point is seen.

▶ Bowel ischemia: poor mural enhancement, segmental mesenteric edema, and pneumatosis. Non-enhancing bowel wall is a highly specific sign of ischemia. Intraluminal stone should not be present.

Teaching Points

Gallstone ileus occurs more frequently in women of advanced age, commonly in the setting of chronic cholecystitis. It manifests as mechanical bowel obstruction with symptoms of abdominal pain, nausea, vomiting, fever, and abdominal distention. Rigler's triad, which consists of small bowel obstruction, gas in biliary tract, and an ectopic obstructing gallstone, is the classic finding, but is rarely identified prospectively on abdominal radiographs.. On CT, a biliary-enteric fistula is often identified and the impacted gallstone, which is usually laminated and large (more than 2.5 cm), is usually identified with certainty. Such stones typically lodge at narrow points of the GI tract, including the duodenum, ligament of Treitz, ileocecal valve, and sigmoid colon. The impaction of a gallstone in the duodenum, causing gastric outlet obstruction, is referred to as Bouveret syndrome.

Management

Surgery is indicated to relieve the mechanical bowel obstruction and to excise the gallbladder and associated biliary-enteric fistula.

Further Reading

1. Reimann A, Yeh BM, Breiman RS, Joe BN, Qayyum A, Coakley FV. Atypical cases of gallstone ileus evaluated with multidetector CT. *J Comput Assist Tomogr.* 2004;28(4):523–527.

History

▶ 76-year-old woman with history of porcelain gallbladder on screening CT colonography.

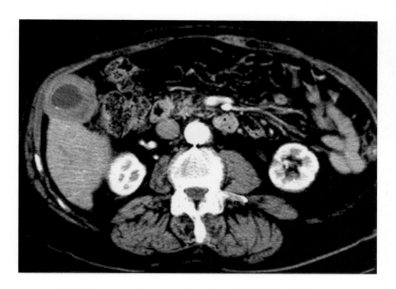

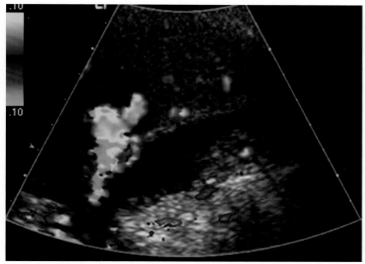

Case 115 Gallbladder Carcinoma

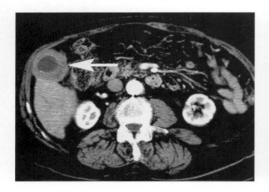 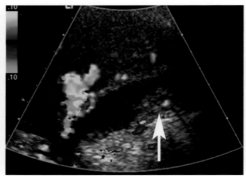

Findings

CT (left) shows marked gallbladder wall thickening (arrow) with heterogeneous enhancement and scattered mural calcifications. Longitudinal color Doppler ultrasound image (right) of the gallbladder shows an irregular, nonmobile, intraluminal soft tissue mass (arrow) with internal vascularity.

Differential Diagnosis

► Chronic cholecystitis: tends to have more symmetric wall thickening and associated gallstones. Xanthogranulomatous cholecystitis is an aggressive form of chronic cholecystitis that may invade adjacent organs and is often indistinguishable from gallbladder carcinoma.

► Adenomyomatosis: diffuse or focal gallbladder wall thickening that has associated ring-down artifact from sludge and stones in Rokitansky-Aschoff sinuses on ultrasound.

Teaching Points

Gallbladder carcinoma has a 4:1 female to male ratio, with peak incidence in the sixth and seventh decades of life. The prevalence of cholelithiasis in patients with gallbladder carcinoma is up to 80 to 90 percent. Earlier reports suggested that porcelain gallbladder is associated with malignant transformation, but more recent pathology series suggest that this association is weak. Imaging findings may be subtle in early-stage disease and are commonly missed. Two percent of patients with gallbladder carcinoma have tumors that are detected incidentally at histopathology after cholecystectomy for stone disease. Imaging findings on sonography and CT include a gallbladder mass replacing the gallbladder, asymmetric wall thickening of the gallbladder wall (focal or diffuse), and a polypoid intraluminal mass usually larger than 1 cm. The appearance may be indistinguishable from chronic cholecystitis. More focal involvement may resemble an area of adenomyomatosis. Involvement of the liver and biliary obstruction is commonly seen at the time of diagnosis. Additional findings suggestive of malignancy include soft tissue infiltration of the hepatoduodenal ligament, extrahepatic biliary obstruction, hepatoduodenal ligament and peripancreatic lymph nodes, encasement of the common hepatic duct, and invasion of the liver and duodenum. Some authors have described bulging of the quadrate lobe of the liver.

Management

Cholecystectomy is performed if there is no tumor extension beyond the gallbladder wall. Extended cholecystectomy and/or partial hepatectomy with regional lymph node dissection may be performed for larger tumors or those that infiltrate the porta hepatis.

Further Reading

1. Levy AD, Murakata LA, Rohrmann CA Jr. Gallbladder carcinoma: radiologic-pathologic correlation. *RadioGraphics*. 2001;*21*(2):295–314.

History

▶ 42-year-old woman with nausea, abdominal pain, and fever after recent cholecystectomy.

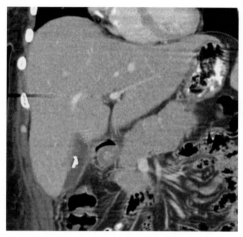

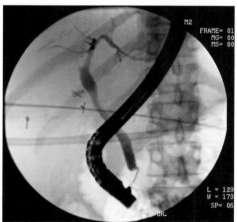

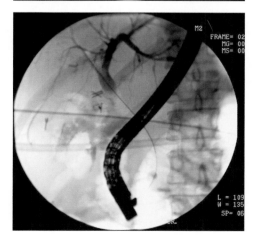

Case 116 Post-cholecystectomy bile leak

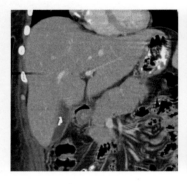 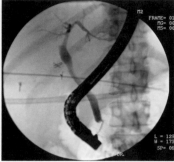 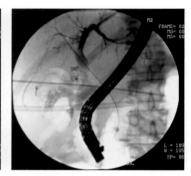

Findings

CT (left) shows a low-density fluid collection, suggestive of biloma, surrounding cholecystectomy clips in the gallbladder fossa. A follow-up ERCP (center and right) shows contrast extravasation from the cystic duct stump into the gallbladder fossa.

Differential Diagnosis

▶ Abscess: infected post-operative fluid collections are not reliably distinguished from sterile ones at imaging, but abscesses often have rim enhancement. Adjacent fat stranding or gas within the fluid suggests abscess. Suspected abscesses should be evaluated carefully for dropped gallstones, which may be a nidus of infection.

▶ Hematoma: typically higher CT density than a biloma and may contain a hematocrit level.

Teaching Points

Laparoscopic cholecystectomy has a higher rate of bile leak than open cholecystectomy. In most cases, the bile leak is from the cystic duct stump. Other sites of bile leak include injury to intra- or extrahepatic ducts and anomalous ducts that previously drained the liver directly into the gallbladder (ducts of Luschka). CT is often the first imaging modality used to identify the leak; ERCP is helpful in further evaluation to identify the source of the leak.

Management

Many bile leaks resolve spontaneously after percutaneous drainage of the biloma. A minority of cases require endoscopic treatment such as placement of a temporary stent across the injured ducts. More complicated biliary injuries require surgical repair.

Further Readings

1. Choi JY, Kim MJ, Park MS, Kim JH, Lim JS, Oh YT, et al. Imaging findings of biliary and nonbiliary complications following laparoscopic surgery. *European Radiology*. 2006; *16*:1906–1914.
2. Wright TB, Bertino RB, Bishop AF, Brady TM, Castaneda F, Berkman WA, et al. Complications of laparoscopic cholecystectomy and their interventional radiologic management. *RadioGraphics*. 1993; *13*:119–128.

History

▶ 49-year-old man with acute right upper quadrant pain and white blood cell count of 18,000.

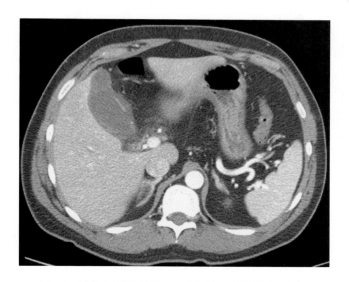

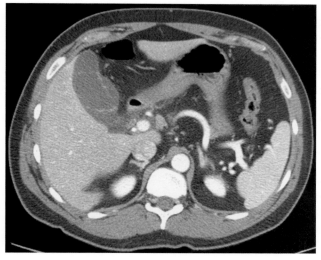

Case 117 Gangrenous Cholecystitis

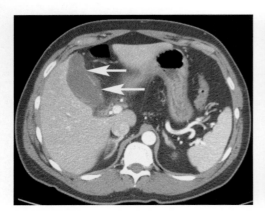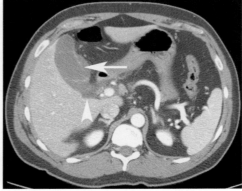

Findings

CT images show a dilated gallbladder with mural thickening, discontinuous mural enhancement (arrows), and pericholecystic fluid (arrowhead). No gallstones are present.

Differential Diagnosis

▶ Uncomplicated acute cholecystitis: mural thickening with diffuse uninterrupted mural enhancement similar in brightness to the liver parenchyma.
▶ Duodenitis: inflammatory stranding and mural thickening centers on the affected bowel.
▶ Benign gallbladder edema: secondary to portal hypertension or hypoproteinemia. Absence of focal tenderness (sonographic Murphy's sign).
▶ Gallbladder carcinoma: may appear as eccentric gallbladder wall thickening and show invasion of adjacent liver and enlarged regional lymph nodes.

Teaching Points

Gangrenous cholecystitis is associated with a higher morbidity and mortality rate than typical acute cholecystitis. Risk factors include old age, cardiovascular disease, and white blood cell count above 17,000. Clinically, gangrenous cholecystitis may be difficult to distinguish from uncomplicated cholecystitis. The classic ultrasound findings of cholecystitis are less commonly present in complicated forms, with approximately one-third of patients having a negative sonographic Murphy sign. Ultrasound may demonstrate irregular gallbladder wall thickening, intraluminal membranes, or intramural gas. CT can be accurate in identifying gangrenous cholecystitis, with defects in wall perfusion (interruptions in wall enhancement) representing the most sensitive finding in recent studies of CT and MRI. Other findings include increased short axis diameter, intraluminal membranes, intramural air, and lack of gallstones (acalculous cholecystitis).

Management

Gangrenous gallbladders may be challenging to resect laparoscopically and may require conversion to an open procedure. Cholecystostomy drainage is a suitable alternative in those patients who are not good surgical candidates.

Further Readings

1. WuCH, Chen CC, Wang CJ, Wong YC, Wang LJ, Huang CC, Lo WC, Chen HW. Discrimination of gangrenous from uncomplicated acute cholecystitis: accuracy of CT findings. *Abdom Imaging*. 2011 Apr;36(2):174–8.
2. Singh AK, Sagar P. Gangrenous cholecystitis: prediction with CT imaging. *Abdom Imaging*. 2005 Mar-Apr;*30*(2):218–221.

History

▶ 50-year-old woman with episodic but acutely worsening right upper quadrant pain.

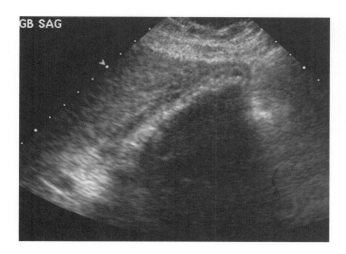

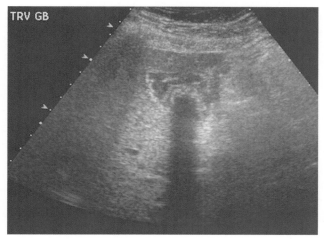

Case 118 Acute cholecystitis

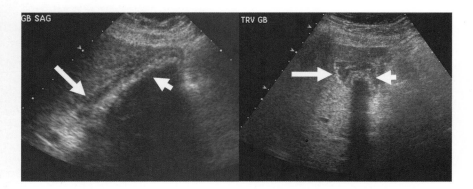

Findings

Ultrasound images of the gallbladder show diffuse mural thickening (long arrows) and multiple calculi (short arrows) that produce posterior acoustic shadowing. Right upper quadrant pain was elicited by pushing on the gallbladder with the ultrasound transducer (positive sonographic Murphy sign).

Differential Diagnosis

► Secondary gallbladder thickening: may occur in a variety of liver or systemic disorders such as hypoproteinemia or portal hypertension. A sonographic Murphy sign should be absent.
► Chronic cholecystitis: may have a similar imaging appearance but patients typically have intermittent or long-standing pain.
► Adenomyomatosis: may cause diffuse or focal gallbladder wall thickening that is associated with "comet tail" artifact from mural cholesterol deposition and small cystic spaces in the areas of wall thickening.

Teaching Points

Acute cholecystitis develops in the setting of biliary stasis and is commonly due to an obstructing gallstone in the gallbladder neck or cystic duct. Less commonly, acalculous cholecystitis occurs when viscous sludge that forms in the setting of biliary dysmotility related to a prolonged fasting state and/or medications serves as a source of obstruction. The ultrasound findings of gallstones with a positive sonographic Murphy sign (focal right upper quadrant pain induced by pressing on the gallbladder using the ultrasound transducer) or gallbladder mural thickening (more than 3mm) have positive predictive values that exceed 92 percent. Conversely, a sonographically normal gallbladder with an absent Murphy sign has a negative predictive value that approaches 100 percent. Mural hyperemia and gallbladder distension (more than 10cm in long axis) are other sonographic findings in acute cholecystitis. Hepatobiliary scintigraphy may be useful if the sonographic findings are equivocal. It is important to note that diffuse gallbladder mural thickening is not specific to cholecystitis and may be seen with a variety of liver diseases or systemic processes.

Management

Acute cholecystitis is usually treated with elective cholecystectomy after a course of antibiotic therapy. Percutaneous cholecystostomy may be performed in poor surgical candidates.

Further Reading

1. van Breda Vriesman AC, Engelbrecht MR, Smithuis RHM, et al. Diffuse gallbladder wall thickening: differential diagnosis. *Am. J. Roentgenol.* 2007; 188: 495–501.

History

▶ 60-year-old woman with diabetes mellitus now has worsening right upper quadrant pain.

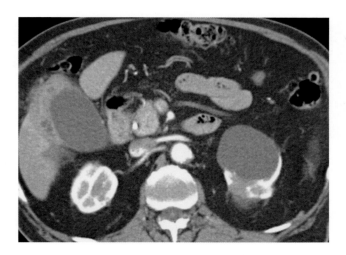

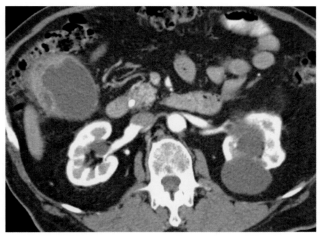

Case 119 Xanthogranulomatous Cholecystitis

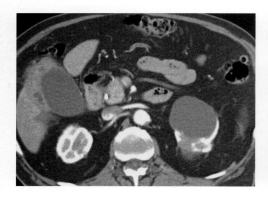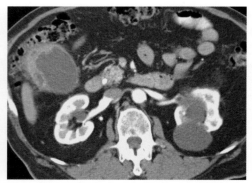

Findings

Intravenous contrast-enhanced CT image shows distension of the gallbladder and marked thickening (arrow) of the gallbladder fundus with extension of the thickening into the adjacent liver. There is adjacent fat stranding and multiple irregular hypoattenuating foci within the thickened gallbladder wall.

Differential Diagnosis

▶ Gallbladder adenocarcinoma: may be indistinguishable from xanthogranulomatous cholecystitis, especially when there is invasion of the adjacent liver or extension of the inflammatory process into the adjacent fat.
▶ Metastasis: gallbladder is an uncommon location for metastatic disease but can be seen in patients with melanoma. Metastases to the gallbladder mimic gallbladder carcinoma, producing infiltrating or polypoid lesions.
▶ Adenomyomatosis: focal or diffuse gallbladder wall thickening, particularly at the gallbladder fundus, and often with small cystic foci. No infiltration of the liver or fat stranding.

Teaching Points

Xanthogranulomatous cholecystitis is an unusual, severe form of chronic cholecystitis that occurs most often in older women. Most patients complain of right upper quadrant pain and vomiting and have a positive sonographic Murphy sign. The imaging findings are similar to those of gallbladder carcinoma: a thick gallbladder wall with indistinct or infiltrative margins and extension of the process into the adjacent liver, surrounding fat, and in some cases adjacent bowel. Characteristic irregular low-attenuation foci in the gallbladder wall are suggestive of the diagnosis. These low-attenuation foci represent lipid-laden xanthogranulomatous inflammation. Gallstones, disruption of the mucosal line, pericholecystic fluid, and bile duct dilatation may also be present. The hypoattenuating intramural cystic foci are hypoechoic when seen on sonography.

Management

Xanthogranulomatous cholecystitis is surgically excised. It is difficult to distinguish xanthogranulomatous cholecystitis from gallbladder adenocarcinoma at preoperative imaging.

Further Readings

1. Levy AD, Murakata LA, Abbott RM, Rohrmann CA, Jr. From the archives of the AFIP. Benign tumors and tumorlike lesions of the gallbladder and extrahepatic bile ducts: radiologic-pathologic correlation. Armed Forces Institute of Pathology. *RadioGraphics*. 2002;*22*(2):387–413.
2. Levy AD, Murakata LA, Rohrmann CA, Jr. Gallbladder carcinoma: radiologic-pathologic correlation. *RadioGraphics*. 2001;*21*(2):295–314.

Part 9

Bile Ducts

History:

► 56-year-old man with upper abdominal discomfort and jaundice.

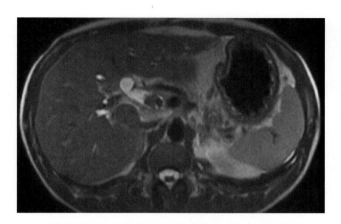

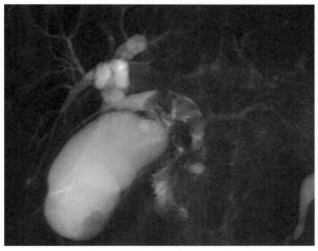

Case 120 Choledocholithiasis

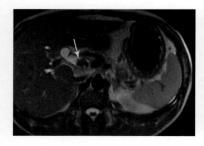 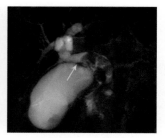

Findings

T2-weighted MRI (left) shows multiple T2 hypointense filling defects (arrow) dependently located within in the common bile duct consistent with calculi. MRCP (right) shows multiple filling defects (arrow) in the common bile duct and moderate intrahepatic duct dilatation.

Differential Diagnosis

- ▶ Pneumobilia: air bubbles are also T2 hypointense filling defects but would be nondependent within the bile duct.
- ▶ Hemobilia: usually post procedural.
- ▶ Flow artifacts: filling defects typically located centrally in the bile duct and inconsistently seen on all sequences.

Teaching Points

Choledocholithiasis is the most common cause of biliary tract obstruction. Ultrasound is a readily available, noninvasive imaging modality often used as the initial investigation of choice for biliary disease. MRCP is extremely sensitive (81 to100 percent) and specific (92 to 100 percent) for gallstones and also provides excellent anatomic definition of the biliary tract. MRCP also has the advantage of being a noninvasive test without exposure to ionizing radiation. ERCP has a similar sensitivity and specificity when compared with MRCP, but the former requires sedation, exposure to ionizing radiation, and carries a risk of pancreatitis or cholangitis (5 to 8 percent). Endoscopic ultrasound has a similar sensitivity (87 to 98 percent) to MRCP; however, this is a relatively invasive procedure requiring sedation.

Management

If an obstructing calculus requiring intervention is shown on ultrasound, ERCP may be more appropriate than MRCP, as this allows the possibility of decompression by sphincterotomy, stone extraction, and stent placement. Because of the risk of inducing pancreatitis, ERCP is recommended over the noninvasive imaging techniques when the need for intervention is considered probable. If this does not relieve the obstruction, laparoscopic or open cholecystectomy with common bile duct exploration may be required. MRCP is the test of choice in patients with low to moderate suspicion of CBD stones.

Further Readings

1. Freitas ML, Bell RL, et al. Choledocholithiasis: evolving standards for diagnosis and management. World J Gastroenterol. 2006; *12*(20):3162–3167.
2. Holm AN and Gerke H. What should be done with a dilated bile duct? *Curr Gastroenterol Rep.* 2010;*12*(2):150–156.
3. Verma D, Kapadia A, et al. EUS vs. MRCP for detection of choledocholithiasis. *Gastrointest Endosc.* 2006;*64*(2):248–254.

History

▶ 40-year-old woman with abdominal pain.

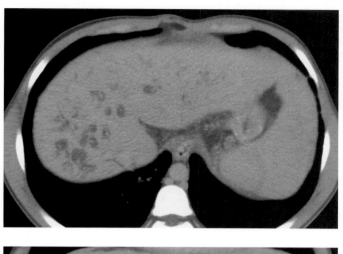

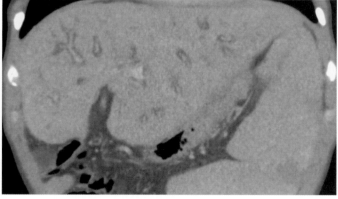

Case 121 Caroli Disease

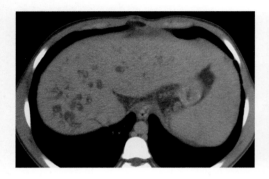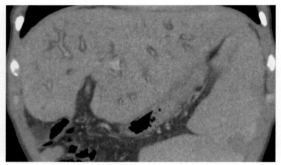

Findings

Axial and coronal CT images show numerous round intrahepatic cystic lesions communicating with the bile ducts. Enhancing portal radicals are present within the cysts.

Differential Diagnosis

▶ Primary sclerosing cholangitis: typically demonstrates isolated fusiform bile duct dilatation, rather than saccular dilatation. Characterized by multiple intra- and extrahepatic strictures, caudate lobe enlargement, and a lobulated liver contour. Seventy percent of patients have inflammatory bowel disease.

▶ Recurrent pyogenic cholangitis: typically demonstrates central fusiform bile duct dilatation with peripheral tapering, rather than saccular dilatation. Hepatolithiasis is almost always present.

▶ Polycystic liver disease: may present with both renal and hepatic cysts. Typically intra- and extrahepatic bile ducts are normal, and hepatic cysts do not demonstrate ductal communication.

Teaching Points

Caroli disease is a rare autosomal recessive disorder resulting from abnormal intrahepatic bile ductal development. Two types have been described: Caroli disease and Caroli syndrome (Caroli disease with hepatic fibrosis). Caroli disease occurs following arrested ductal plate remodeling of the larger intrahepatic ducts. Caroli syndrome occurs with further arrested remodeling later in embryogenesis, during development of the remaining more peripheral biliary ducts. Caroli disease typically manifests as saccular or fusiform cystic intrahepatic ductal dilatation. Sludge or stones may develop within the dilated bile ducts. Irregular walls and strictures may be present. On CT, these hypoattenuating lesions typically demonstrate central enhancing fibrovascular bundles within the cystic intrahepatic ducts ("central dot sign"). T2-weighted MR and MRCP show communication between the cystic dilatations and the bile ducts. Complications in Caroli disease include cholangitis, liver abscess formation, bilirubin stone formation, cholangiocarcinoma, and obstruction. In Caroli syndrome, cirrhosis and portal venous hypertension are often present at the time of presentation. Associated conditions include renal cystic diseases such as medullary sponge kidney.

Management

In patients with disease that results in either repeated episodes of cholangitis or acquired biliary cirrhosis, orthotopic liver transplantation is preferable.

Further Reading

1. Levy AD, Rohrmann CA, Murakata LA, et al. Caroli Disease: Radiologic Spectrum with Pathologic Correlation. *Am J Roentgenol.* 2002; *179*: 1053–1057.

History

▶ 33-year-old woman with right upper quadrant pain.

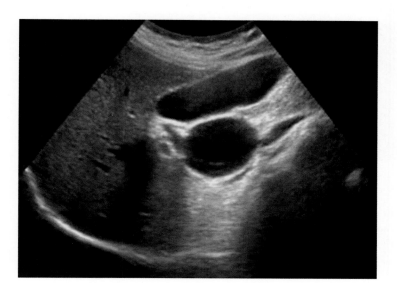

Case 122 Choledochal cyst, Type 1

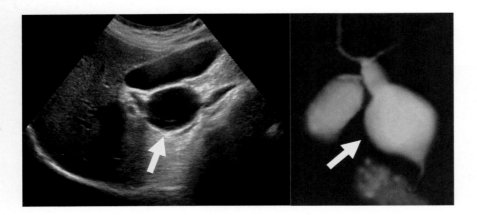

Findings

Ultrasound and MRCP (right) show marked, saccular dilatation of the extrahepatic common bile duct (arrow) without an obstructing lesion and no evidence of intrahepatic bile duct dilatation.

Differential Diagnosis

▶ Obstructed common bile duct: would not cause the profound and focal biliary dilatation seen in the present case and there should be intrahepatic duct dilatation.

▶ Pancreatic pseudocyst: may mimic choledochal cyst on US and require additional imaging to depict it as separate from the extrahepatic bile duct.

Teaching Points

Choledochal cyst is a nonhereditary congenital dilatation of the extrahepatic bile duct, which may have intrahepatic duct involvement in the most severe cases. It is thought to be caused by reflux of pancreatic secretions into the common bile duct because of an anomalous pancreaticobiliary junction. The majority of patients with choledochal cysts (80 percent) are diagnosed in childhood and are female (4:1). Five types of choledochal cysts have been described by Todani et al: segmental saccular or fusiform dilatation of the extrahepatic bile duct (type 1, most common); an extrahepatic bile duct diverticulum (type 2); ectatic intraduodenal segment of the extrahepatic bile duct (type 3, a choledochocele); multifocal saccular dilatations of the extrahepatic and intrahepatic bile ducts (type 4); and multifocal segmental dilatation of the intrahepatic bile duct only (Caroli disease). Imaging shows fusiform or saccular dilatation of the bile ducts. Patients present with symptoms related to biliary stasis, such as RUQ pain, fever, and jaundice, and have a 15 percent risk for the development of cholangiocarcinoma, which may occur in young adulthood. This increased risk of cholangiocarcinoma remains after surgical treatment, particularly after incomplete resection, indicating the need for lifelong surveillance. Multiple simple renal parenchymal cysts and renal tubular ectasia (medullary sponge kidney) are associated anomalies.

Management

Patients with a newly detected choledochal cyst should be recommended for gastroenterology referral as a prelude to possible surgical resection given the risk of malignant degeneration.

Further Reading

1. Mortelé KJ, Rocha TC, Streeter JL, et al. Multimodality imaging of pancreatic and biliary congenital anomalies. *RadioGraphics* 2006; *26*:715–773.

History

▶ 42-year-old man with history of ulcerative colitis, elevated liver function tests, and prior instrumentation.

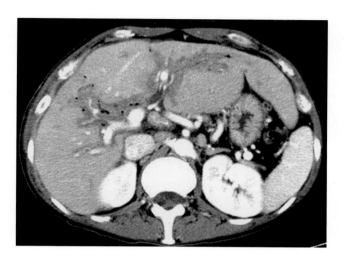

Case 123 Primary Sclerosing Cholangitis

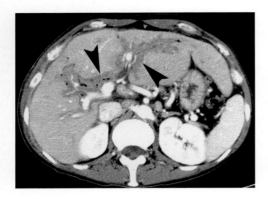

Findings

CT with intravenous contrast shows extensive periportal edema (arrowheads) associated with pneumobilia, which is a result of prior instrumentation. The pneumobilia shows the caliber of the bile ducts is small to minimally dilated to the periphery of the liver.

Differential Diagnosis

- ► Recurrent pyogenic cholangitis: typically occurs in patients from Asia and is associated with intrahepatic stones, usually with dilated bile ducts.
- ► Cholangiocarcinoma: bile duct dilatation almost always present in central tumors.
- ► Ascending cholangitis: usually has prior biliary disease or obstruction and generally not associated with inflammatory bowel disease.

Teaching Points

Primary sclerosing cholangitis is a chronic progressive inflammatory disorder that is more common in men and middle-aged persons with a mean age of 39 years, and is associated with inflammatory bowel disease in approximately 75 percent of cases. The long-term sequelae of primary sclerosing cholangitis are cirrhosis, portal hypertension, and ultimately liver failure, usually occurring within 10 years. Though not the preferred imaging modality for evaluating primary sclerosing cholangitis, ultrasound can reveal thickening of common bile duct wall with or without luminal obliteration. At CT, one may see a beaded appearance of the biliary tract or mildly dilated discrete segments of intrahepatic ducts that may extend close to the liver periphery. Dilation of the extrahepatic biliary system is usually absent, but there may be common duct stenosis as well as mural thickening, periportal edema, and biliary nodularity and enhancement. At MRCP, mild irregular intrahepatic ductal dilation with a beaded appearance without expected side branch dilation, which is known as "pruning," is often seen. Sclerosing cholangitis predisposes patients to develop cholangiocarcinoma.

Management

Repeated mechanical balloon dilatation of affected bile ducts may be attempted at ERCP. Imaging surveillance may be utilized to screen for cholangiocarcinoma.

Further Reading

1. Yeh BM, Liu PS, Soto JA, Corvera CA and Hussain HK. MR imaging and CT of the biliary tract. *RadioGraphics*. 2009. *29*(6): 1669–1688.

History

▶ 38-year-old HIV-positive man with pruritus, diarrhea, and abnormal liver function tests.

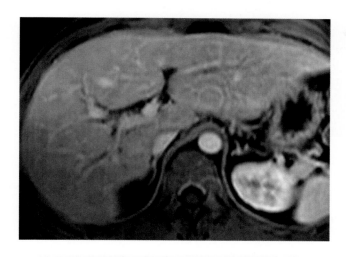

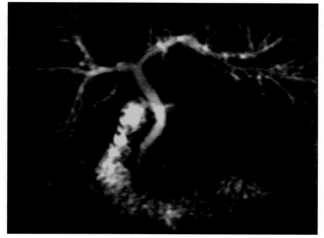

Case 124 AIDS Cholangiopathy

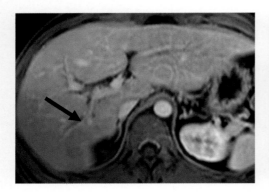 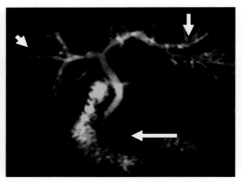

Findings

T1-weighted MR image obtained during the portal venous phase shows mild intrahepatic bile duct dilation (black arrow). MRCP image shows numerous intrahepatic bile duct strictures (short white arrows) with associated mild bile duct dilation and a stricture at the ampullary portion of the distal common bile duct (long white arrow).

Differential Diagnosis

▶ Primary sclerosing cholangitis: intra- and extrahepatic bile duct stricturing and dilation, often with a beaded appearance. Papillary strictures are typically absent.

▶ Distal cholangiocarcinoma: may manifest as a distal common bile duct stricture. Associated intrahepatic strictures would be rare.

Teaching Points

Opportunistic biliary tract infections by several organisms have been implicated in the development of AIDS-related cholangitis but not directly demonstrated as causative. Direct involvement by the HIV virus has also been postulated as an etiology. Four patterns of AIDS-related cholangiopathy have been reported: (1) papillary stenosis with dilatation of bile ducts and delayed drainage; (2) sclerosing cholangitis characterized by focal strictures and dilatation of the intra and/or extrahepatic bile ducts; (3) combined papillary stenosis and intra and/or extrahepatic sclerosing cholangitis, and (4) long extrahepatic bile duct strictures. US findings also include dilatation and mural thickening of the gallbladder and common bile duct as well as pericholecystic fluid. Dilated intrahepatic ducts, gallbladder dilatation and sludge are also commonly found. On CT, inflammation of the gallbladder or bile ducts is manifest by wall thickening and/or abnormal contrast enhancement. Direct cholangiography and MRCP are more sensitive and specific than CT and US in depicting the mural irregularity of the extrahepatic ducts that result from exuberant periductal inflammation, mucosal ulcers, and interstitial edema of AIDS-related cholangitis.

Management

AIDS cholangiopathy once carried a very grave prognosis. Highly active antiretroviral therapy has made AIDS cholangiopathy uncommon. Strictures can be managed with stenting. High serum alkaline phosphatase level is associated with a worse outcome.

Further Reading

1. Vermani N, Kang M, Khandelwal N, et al. MR cholangiopancreatographic demonstration of biliary tract abnormalities in AIDS-cholangiopathy: report of two cases. *Clin Radiol.* 2009; *64*:335–338.

History

► 53-year-old man with known primary sclerosing cholangitis (PSC), complains of abdominal pain and fevers.

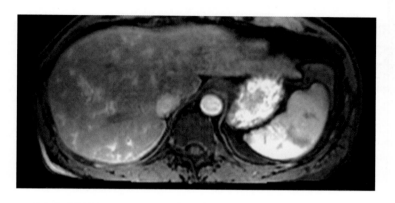

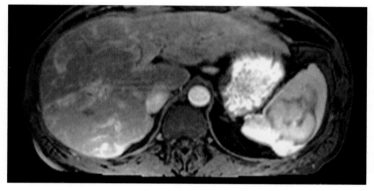

Case 125   Acute Cholangitis

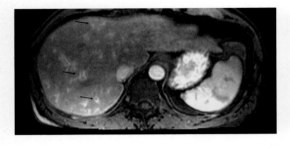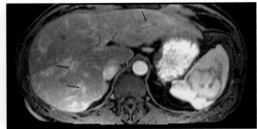

Findings

Two contiguous T1-weighted fat-saturated images following intravenous gadolinium demonstrate multifocal areas of mild intrahepatic duct dilatation consistent with the patient's known PSC. In addition there is marked hyperenhancement of the wall of multiple intrahepatic ducts (arrows) and mild hyperemia in the surrounding liver parenchyma.

Differential Diagnosis

► Primary sclerosing cholangitis: this appearance can be seen in uncomplicated PSC, and the diagnosis of acute cholangitis is based on the clinical and laboratory findings.

Teaching Points

Acute cholangitis is inflammation of the biliary ductal system, usually secondary to biliary obstruction, although it may also be secondary to instrumentation of the biliary tree for percutaneous transhepatic cholangiography (PTC) or endoscopic retrograde cholangiopancreatography (ERCP). The function of imaging is primarily to confirm the presence of biliary obstruction and to determine the underlying cause. CT and MRCP can provide more information about the site and cause of any obstruction. Biliary duct dilatation is extremely common. Contrast-enhanced CT demonstrates transient parenchymal enhancement in the liver in a periportal distribution. MRCP may show thickening of the walls of the bile ducts with increased enhancement of the wall. Wedge shaped areas of high T2 signal and hyperenhancement in a periportal distribution may also be seen.

Management

Patients are frequently septic; however, many respond well to antibiotics and rehydration. Patients who do not respond to these measures require urgent decompression of the biliary tree using ERCP, PTC or open surgical drainage. ERCP has become the treatment of choice because it is superior to PTC in terms of avoiding morbidity and mortality. However, PTC may be necessary in cases where ERCP is not possible, for example when there has been prior surgery which renders the ampulla of Vater inaccessible. Open surgery is rarely the first-line treatment but may be utilized when ERCP and PTC have failed.

Further Reading

1. Watanabe Y, Nagayama M, et al. MR imaging of acute biliary disorders. *RadioGraphics*. 2007; *27*(2):477–495

History

▶ 87-year-old woman with painless jaundice and weight loss.

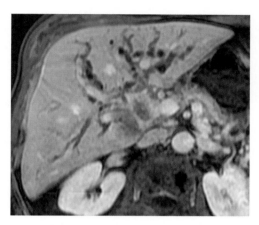

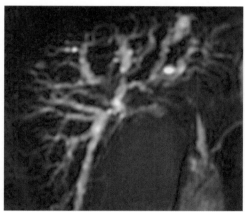

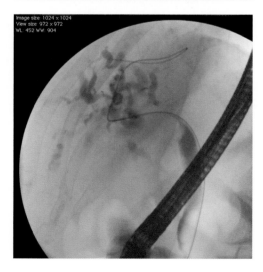

Case 126 Hilar (Klatskin) Cholangiocarcinoma

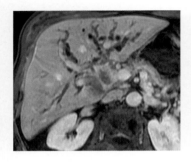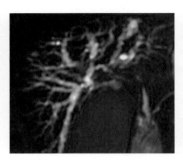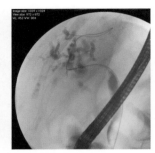

Findings

T1-weighted MR obtained in the portal venous phase (left) shows an ill-defined hypovascular infiltrative mass arising near the confluence of the main right and left bile ducts, causing moderate intrahepatic bile duct dilatation. MRCP (center) shows dilated intrahepatic bile ducts and a normal distal common bile duct and pancreatic duct, confirming the level of obstruction at the level of the hepatic hilum. ERCP (right) obtained during stent placement demonstrates moderate intrahepatic dilatation and a normal-caliber common bile duct.

Differential Diagnosis

► Pancreatic carcinoma: arises from ductal epithelium of the exocrine pancreas, causes abrupt obstruction and dilatation of the main pancreatic duct and distal CBD, and can infiltrate the peripancreatic fat.
► Primary sclerosing cholangitis (PSC): mild dilatation of both intra- and extrahepatic bile ducts, often with isolated obstruction of segmental intrahepatic bile ducts. ERCP images show irregular biliary strictures, beading and pruning.
► Other porta hepatis tumor: hepatocellular carcinoma, lymphoma, and hilar liver metastasis (breast or gastrointestinal cancers) may invade and obstruct the central intrahepatic bile ducts.

Teaching Points

Cholangiocarcinoma is an adenocarcinoma that arises from bile duct epithelium. Cholangiocarcinoma is usually classified as either intrahepatic (peripheral) or extrahepatic. When the malignancy arises from one of the hepatic ducts or the bifurcation of the common hepatic duct, it is called hilar cholangiocarcinoma, or Klatskin tumor. These three different types of cholangiocarcinoma—extrahepatic distal, peripheral intrahepatic, and hilar—are traditionally regarded as distinct disease entities clinically, therapeutically, and radiologically. The most typical presentation of hilar cholangiocarcinoma is as a periductal infiltrating mass (over 70 percent of cases). About 80 percent of these tumors are hyperattenuating relative to the liver on delayed contrast-enhanced images due to abundant fibrous tissue. Mass-forming and polypoid hilar cholangiocarcinomas are less common. Approximately 20 to 40 percent of patients may undergo surgical resection with curative intent.

Management

Surgical resection including major hepatic resection remains the mainstay of treatment of hilar cholangiocarcinoma. Surgical exploration should only be performed when preoperative examination has shown curative resection to be possible.

Further Reading

1. Han JK, Choi BI, Kim AY, et al. Cholangiocarcinoma: Pictorial Essay of CT and Cholangiographic Findings. *RadioGraphics* 2002; *22*:173–187.

History

► 52-year-old man with mid-epigastric abdominal pain and history of biliary obstruction.

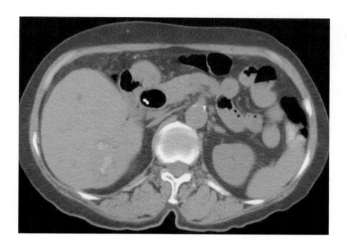

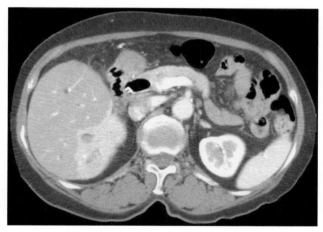

Case 127 Recurrent Pyogenic Cholangitis

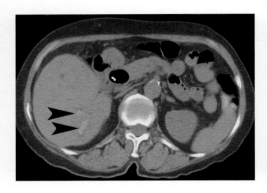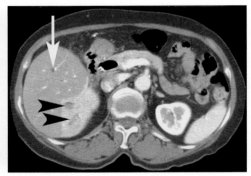

Findings

Axial noncontrast (left) and contrast-enhanced images (right) through the liver show intrahepatic ductal dilatation (arrow) with hyperdense intrahepatic stones (arrowheads).

Differential Diagnosis

▸ Sclerosing cholangitis: Multiple alternating segments of bile duct dilatation and focal strictures, usually associated with inflammatory bowel disease.

▸ Bacterial cholangitis: stones, sludge, and/or pus in bile ducts often associated with prior instrumentation.

▸ cholangiocarcinoma: delayed contrast-enhancement within infiltrating parenchymal mass.

Teaching Points

Recurrent pyogenic cholangitis, (a.k.a. oriental cholangiohepatitis or intrahepatic pigment stone disease) is endemic to South Asian countries and associated with recurrent bouts of fever, chills, abdominal pain and jaundice. Cholangitis due to enteric organisms such as *E.coli* is most common, though parasites such as the roundworm *Ascaris lumbricorum* or liver fluke *Clonorchis* may also be involved. Biliary stasis is thought to contribute to the characteristic development of intraductal biliary sludge, putty-like biliary pigment stones, biliary abscesses, and bile duct dilatation and strictures. Biliary stones are typically in the bile ducts rather than the gallbladder. With time, lobar or segmental liver volume loss is seen with distortion of the liver contour and biliary architecture. The extent of liver parenchymal atrophy can be profound, leaving only dilated ducts surrounded by fibrous scar tissue. Biliary stones may be high-attenuation or isodense to liver, and should not enhance with intravenous contrast material. Ultrasound can miss small stones and ductal dilatation due to biliary gas or debris. Biliary gas is commonly seen in these patients due to prior interventions including sphincterotomy. Associated splenomegaly may result from obliteration of portal vein branches and liver fibrosis. The disease predisposes to cholangiocarcinoma.

Management

Treatment is with intravenous antibiotics and mechanical decompression of the biliary system by ERCP with sphincterotomy and/or percutaneous transhepatic cholangiography. Surgical approaches include choledochostomy, removal of stones, T-tube placement, and potentially partial hepatectomy.

Further Reading

1. Kim JH, Kim TK, Eun HW, Byun JY, Lee MG, Ha HK, Auh YH. CT findings of cholangiocarcinoma associated with recurrent pyogenic cholangitis. *Am J Roentgenol.* 2006; *187*(6): 1571–1577.

History

▶ 37-year-old man presenting with right upper quadrant pain.

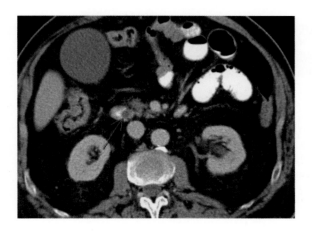

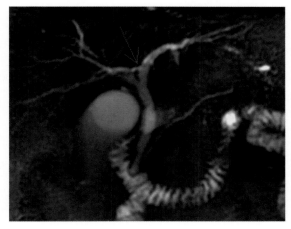

Case 128 Choledochocele

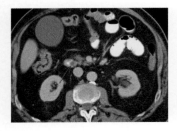 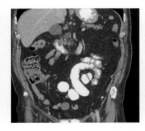 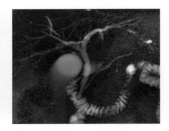

Findings

CT images show a round, low-density abnormality projecting into the lumen of the duodenum at the level of the ampulla of Vater. There is no biliary or pancreatic ductal dilatation. An oblique coronal thick slab MRCP image (right image) confirms the location of the finding, and shows that the cystic structure arises from telescoping of the common bile duct into the duodenal lumen.

Differential Diagnosis

▶ Gastrointestinal duplication cyst: lacks communication to the common bile duct. Only 5 percent occur in the duodenum, with the majority located in the remainder of the small bowel.

▶ Intraductal papillary mucinous tumor: will have lobulated or pleomorphic shape. Does not commonly protrude into the duodenal lumen. Typically connects to the pancreatic duct.

▶ Bulging papilla due to impacted stone: will display inflamed papilla with homogeneous enhancement greater than that of the duodenal mucosa.

Teaching Points

Choledochal cysts are rare congenital biliary tract anomalies characterized by biliary tree dilatation. Todani Type 3 choledochal cysts, or choledochoceles, account for 5 percent of all bile duct cysts but are not embryologically related to the cystic dilatations of other choledochal cysts. Choledochoceles appear as a protrusion of a focally dilated intramural segment of distal common bile duct (CBD) into the duodenum. Patients can present with intermittent biliary colic, jaundice, and recurrent pancreatitis. However, many choledochal cysts are detected incidentally without symptoms referring to the biliary tract. A choledochocele alone can cause cholecystitis or cholangitis. MRCP, CT, and cholangiography may show a rounded dilatation of the terminal bile duct that protrudes into the duodenal lumen.

Management

In symptomatic patients, choledochoceles may be successfully managed with endoscopic sphincterotomy, surgical excision, or both. Endoscopic sphincterotomy and surveillance can be performed in asymptomatic patients, as there is a reported risk of biliary malignancy that is lower than with other types of choledochal cysts.

Further Readings

1. Mortelé KJ, Rocha TC, Streeter JL, Taylor AJ. Multimodality imaging of pancreatic and biliary congenital anomalies. *RadioGraphics*. 2006; *26*: 715–731.
2. Yu J, Turner MA, Fulcher AS. Congenital anomalies and normal variants of the pancreaticobiliary tract and pancreas in adults: part I, biliary tract. *Am J Roentgenol*. 2005; *25*: 1299–1320.

History

▶ 65-year-old man with history of colon cancer and prior cholecystectomy, presents with jaundice.

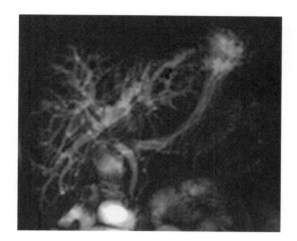

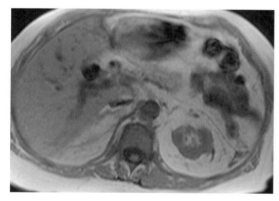

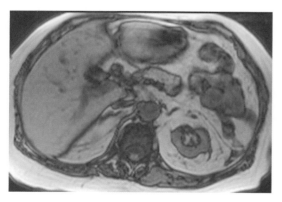

Case 129 Benign Bile Duct Stricture (Post-Cholecystectomy)

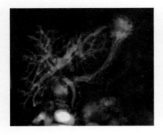 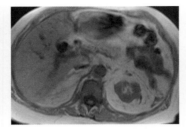 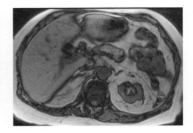

Findings

MRCP (left image) shows marked intrahepatic bile duct dilatation. The common bile duct is only mildly dilated, measuring 7 mm. There is a 1.5 cm tight stricture at the hepatic hilum. The T1-weighted image with longer echo time (in-phase image, center) shows blooming due to susceptibility artifact in the approximate location of the stricture (when compared to the out-of-phase image, right). The gallbladder and cystic duct are not visualized.

Differential Diagnosis

▶ Other benign bile duct strictures: may occur from acute or chronic pancreatitis, following passage of a stone, in patients with primary sclerosing cholangitis or recurrent pyogenic cholangitis, and from idiopathic causes (30 percent)

▶ Malignant stricture: extrahepatic cholangiocarcinoma, metastases, and lymphoma can cause bile duct strictures. Malignant strictures are typically more irregularly bordered, asymmetric in appearance, longer in length, and frequently demonstrate hyperenhancement.

Teaching Points

Benign bile duct strictures tend to be smooth with gradual tapering while an irregular abrupt termination of the bile duct suggests the presence of a malignant stricture. However, there is considerable overlap in these appearances. On CT or MRI, thickening of the bile duct wall with enhancement of the wall suggests the presence of malignancy. Intense and progressive enhancement of a thickened bile duct wall is highly suggestive of a malignant stricture. Primary sclerosing cholangitis is characterized by multifocal structuring and beading of the intra- and extrahepatic biliary tree.

Management

Post-operative strictures may be amenable to percutaneous or endoscopic dilation. In the post-transplant setting however the long-term resolution rate is low (25 percent). Dominant strictures in primary sclerosing cholangitis may cause cholestasis and acute worsening of symptoms. Balloon dilatation may be attempted if the dominant stricture is accessible endoscopically. However, in most cases a single dilatation is not sufficient because of restenosis, and repeated dilatations over years are required. Stenting in these patients has not proven of significant benefit. If endoscopic treatment fails, surgical repair may be attempted. Outcomes are better with distal rather than hilar strictures.

Further Reading

1. Laghi A, Tringali A, et al. Management of hilar biliary strictures. *Am J Gastroenterol.* 2008; *103*(2):458–473.

Part 10   **Pancreas**

History

▶ 37-year-old man with epigastric pain, nausea, and vomiting.

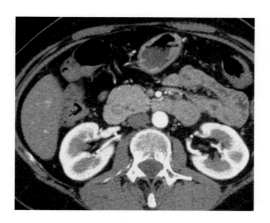

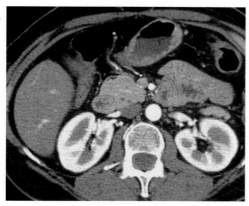

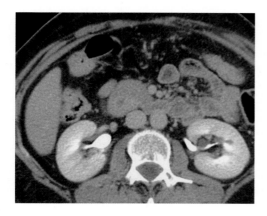

Case 130 Annular Pancreas

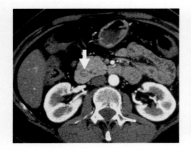 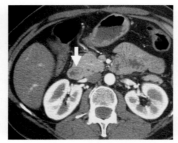 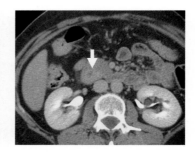

Findings

Serial axial intravenous contrast-enhanced CT images obtained in the arterial phase (left, center) and delayed phase (right) demonstrate pancreatic tissue completely encircling the second part of the duodenum (arrow).

Differential Diagnosis

▶ Duodenal carcinoma: rare malignant tumor, accounting for 1 percent of gastrointestinal tract neoplasms, manifested usually as discrete mass or thickening of the duodenal wall, usually located in the postbulbar portion of the duodenum.

▶ Duodenal hematoma: results from trauma or anticoagulation, causing a focal mass or narrowed lumen with thickened folds with a "picket-fence" pattern.

▶ Pancreatic head carcinoma: ill-defined heterogeneous and hypovascular mass, usually located in the pancreatic head (60 percent). Usually causes pancreatic duct and common bile duct dilatation (double-duct sign) and can be associated with obliteration of the pancreatic fat plane with the superior mesenteric artery or vein, extensive local invasion, and regional lymphadenopathy.

Teaching Points

Annular pancreas is a rare congenital anomaly, with estimated prevalence of one in 2,000 people. Incomplete rotation of the ventral anlage leads to a segment of the pancreas encircling the second part of the duodenum. The encirclement may involve prominent pancreatic tissue, or may be a fibrous band. Annular pancreas can be an isolated finding but can be associated with other congenital abnormalities. In approximately one-half of symptomatic cases, it will manifest in the neonate with gastrointestinal obstruction or bile duct obstruction, possibly associated with pancreatitis. In adults, annular pancreas may be asymptomatic or may cause symptoms of peptic ulcer disease, duodenal obstruction or pancreatitis. There are two types of annular pancreas: the extramural type, in which the ventral pancreatic duct encircles the duodenum to join the main pancreatic duct, or the intramural type, in which the pancreatic tissue is intermingled with muscle fibers in the duodenal wall.

Management

Annular pancreas is considered a developmental anomaly and when confidently diagnosed in an asymptomatic patient can be left alone, avoiding unnecessary surgery.

Further Readings

1. Mortelé KJ, Rocha TC, Streeter JL, et al. Multimodality Imaging of Pancreatic and Biliary Congenital Anomalies. *RadioGraphics*. 2006; *26*:715–731.
2. Jadvar H, Mindelzun RE. Annular Pancreas in Adults: Imaging Features in Seven Patients. *Abdominal Imaging*. 1999; *24*:174–199.

History

▶ 25-year-old woman with recurrent abdominal pain.

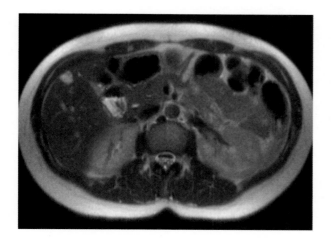

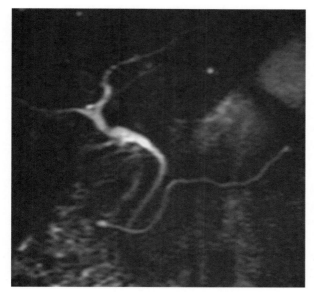

Case 131 Pancreas Divisum

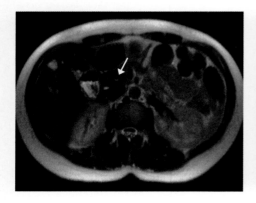 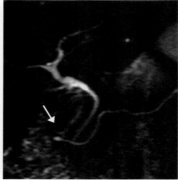

Findings

T2-weighted MRI (left) shows anterior location of the dorsal pancreatic duct (arrow) relative to the common bile duct (CBD) as it courses toward the minor papilla. MRCP (right) shows the dorsal duct crossing the CBD and draining into the minor papilla with cystic dilatation at its point of entry into the minor papilla, consistent with a Santorinicele (arrow).

Differential Diagnosis

▶ Annular pancreas: pancreatic tissue completely or incompletely encircles and narrows the duodenum. The aberrant ventral pancreatic duct communicates with the main pancreatic duct and encircles the duodenum.
▶ Dominant dorsal duct: The dorsal duct is larger in caliber than the ventral duct and it drains via the minor papilla. Normal communication persists between the ventral and dorsal ducts.

Teaching Points

Pancreatic divisum is usually incidentally discovered (9 percent incidence at MRCP or 3 to 8 percent incidence at ERCP). It is the most common variant of the pancreatic ductal system. It occurs from failure of dorsal and the ventral pancreatic buds to fuse in the 7th week of gestation. In pancreas divisum, the dorsal duct drains the majority of the pancreas and the ventral duct drains the inferior head and uncinate process. There are three subtypes: type 1 has no connection between the ventral and dorsal ducts (70 percent); type 2 has an absent ventral duct such that the minor papilla drains the entire pancreas while the major papilla drains the CBD (20 to 25 percent); and type 3 has filamentous or inadequate connection between dorsal and ventral ducts (5 to 6 percent).

Pancreas divisum is found in 12 to 50 percent patients with idiopathic pancreatitis, which is thought to arise because the duct of Santorini (dorsal duct) and minor papilla are too small to drain the secretions of the majority of the pancreas. A Santorinicele can be seen in 15 percent of patients with pancreatic divisum. It is characterized by cystic dilatation of the dorsal duct at the minor papilla.

Management

Sphincterotomy can be performed in patients with pancreatitis. Surgery is reserved for patients with unremitting incapacitating symptoms when conservative measures fail.

Further Reading

1. Soto JA, Lucey BC, Stuhlfaut JW. Pancreas divisum: depiction of multi-row CT. *Radiology* 2005; *235*:503–508.

History

▶ 53-year-old female with longstanding history of alcohol abuse.

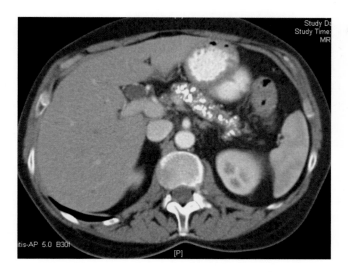

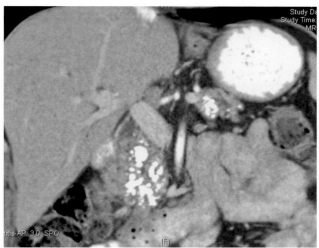

Case 132 Chronic Pancreatitis

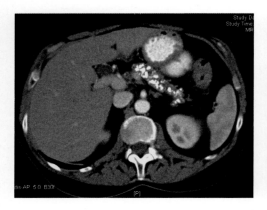 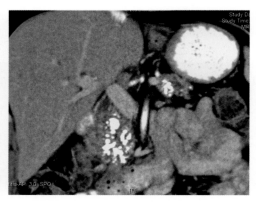

Findings

Contrast-enhanced CT images show coarse and stippled calcifications throughout the pancreas with associated pancreatic atrophy and duct dilation consistent with chronic pancreatitis.

Differential Diagnosis

▶ Islet cell tumors of the pancreas: calcifications tend to be focal, coarse, or irregular, and located centrally within a pancreatic mass.
▶ Intraductal papillary mucinous neoplasm: normal or atrophic parenchyma with side, main, or combined duct dilatation. Dystrophic calcification may be present.

Teaching Points

Chronic pancreatitis is a progressive and chronic inflammatory condition of the pancreas. It is characterised by irreversible fibrosis causing endocrine and exocrine dysfunction. Chronic pancreatitis can cause chronic unremitting abdominal pain, malabsorption, malnutrition and diabetes mellitus. Causes include alcohol, obstruction, stenosis of the papilla, hereditary (autosomal dominant trypsinogen gene mutation) pancreatitis, or idiopathic. On imaging, chronic pancreatitis manifests itself as parenchymal atrophy, dilatation of the main pancreatic duct and its side branches, ductal irregularity with strictures, and intraductal/intraparenchymal calcification. Calcification on CT may be punctate or coarse, and in a focal, segmental or diffuse distribution. These calcifications primarily represent intraductal calculi, either in the main pancreatic duct or in the smaller side branches. Complications include pseudocyst formation which can communicate with the main pancreatic duct, arterial pseudoaneurysm, splenic and portal vein thrombosis, and biliary complications (including common bile duct stones, fistula, and dilatation of the common bile duct due to fibrotic change in the head of the pancreas).

Management

The main focus of management in chronic pancreatitis is to improve pancreatic function, relieve pain, and manage complications. This includes avoiding alcohol, taking supplementary pancreatic enzymes, and getting adequate pain relief. Treatment of blocked ducts from stones may be by stent placement or lithotripsy at endoscopic retrograde cholangio-pancreatography. Surgery is reserved for those in whom conservative treatments fail.

Further Readings

1. Lesniak RJ, Hohenwalter MD, Taylor AJ. Spectrum of causes of pancreatic calcifications. *Am J Roentgenol.* 2002; *178*:79–86.
2. De Backer AI, Mortele KJ, Ros PR et al. Chronic Pancreatitis: diagnostic role of computed tomography and magnetic resonance imaging. *JBR-BTR* 2002; *85*:304–310.

History

▶ 32-year-old woman with severe epigastric pain.

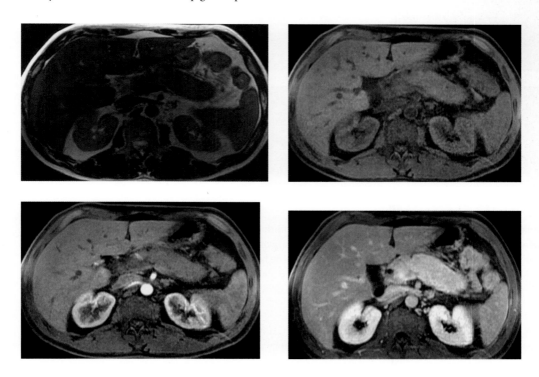

Case 133 Autoimmune Pancreatitis

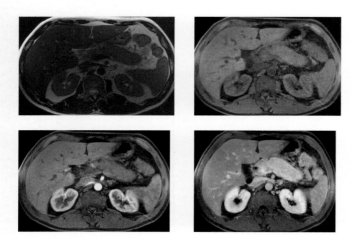

Findings

T2-weighted (top left), T1-weighted (top right), and gadolinium-enhanced early and late phase fat-suppressed T1-weighted MR images show diffuse slight hyperintensity of a "sausage-shaped" pancreas on T2; the gland is hypointense on T1 with diminished enhancement on the late arterial phase and diffuse enhancement on the delayed phase. There is a subtle capsule-like smooth rim of fibrous tissue that is most conspicuous on the T2-weighted and delayed enhanced image. There is no pancreatic or biliary ductal dilation.

Differential Diagnosis

▶ Infiltrative pancreatic adenocarcinoma: aggressive infiltration of malignancy that invades adjacent vessels and organs. Bile duct and pancreatic duct dilation with atrophy of the pancreas distal to the lesion is common.

▶ Acute pancreatitis: characterized by peripancreatic edema and fluid. On MR, the pancreas is heterogeneous hypointense on T1, hyperintense on T2, and variably enhances. There is no surrounding capsule.

▶ Pancreatic lymphoma: focal or diffuse enlargement of the pancreas that is typically hypoattenuating on contrast-enhanced CT, but may have diminished homogenous enhancement. A capsule-like rim has not been described. Regional nodal enlargement may be present.

Teaching Points

Autoimmune pancreatitis is an autoimmune systemic disease that may involve other organs, including bile ducts (80 percent), kidneys (35 percent), salivary glands (15 percent), and the retroperitoneum (10 percent). Elevated serum IgG4 aids in diagnosis. Focal and diffuse patterns occur. Focal autoimmune pancreatitis is often mistaken for pancreatic adenocarcinoma. On CT, autoimmune pancreatitis is characterized by diffuse (40 to 60 percent) or focal (30 to 40 percent) enlargement of the gland with diminished early phase enhancement followed by delayed enhancement. Minimal peripancreatic inflammation and a smooth capsule like rim (12 to 40 percent) may be present. On MR, autoimmune pancreatitis causes featureless (sausage-shaped) pancreatic enlargement with mild T2 hyperintensity and T1 hypointensity. The enhancement patterns on MR are identical to contrast-enhanced CT. The capsule-like rim is T1 and T2 hypointense and has delayed enhancement. Diffuse or segmental narrowing of the main pancreatic duct is characteristic.

Management

Serum IgG4 evaluation or Endoscopic ultrasound with fine needle aspiration is often required for diagnosis. Autoimmune pancreatitis typically resolves following treatment with corticosteroids.

Further Reading

1. Sahani DV, Kalva SP, Farrell J, et al. Autoimmune Pancreatitis: Imaging Findings. *Radiology.* 2004; 233: 345–352.

History

▶ 55-year-old man with chronic epigastric pain and history of alcohol abuse.

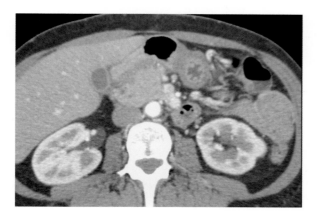

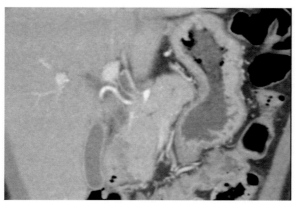

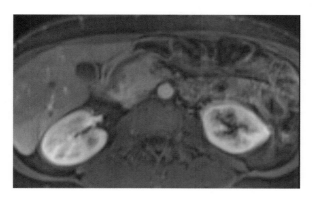

Case 134　Groove Pancreatitis

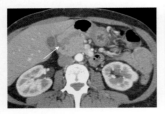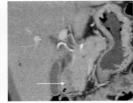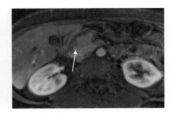

Findings

Axial (left) and coronal (middle) contrast-enhanced CT images shows a sheet-like mass in the region of the groove between the head of the pancreas and the 2nd portion of the duodenum (arrow). It is hypoenhancing relative to the adjacent pancreatic parenchyma. There is no sequela of pancreatitis seen in the head of the pancreas. Gadolinium-enhanced T1-WI obtained in the same patient (right) demonstrates a fibrotic mass in the same region which demonstrates decreased enhancement (arrow).

Differential Diagnosis

► Adenocarcinoma of the head of the pancreas: intrapancreatic, ill-defined mass, similar enhancement characteristics to groove pancreatitis but associated with distal pancreatic duct dilatation, vascular invasion, and localized adenopathy.
► Primary or secondary duodenal neoplasm: intraluminal/submucosal/intramural masses, periduodenal fluid, localized adenopathy, proximal obstruction if intraluminal.
► Cholangiocarcinoma of the distal common bile duct (CBD): irregular stricture of the distal CBD with proximal bile duct dilation.
► Acute pancreatitis of the head of the pancreas: edematous pancreas with abnormal parenchymal signal intensity and enhancement on MRI, peripancreatic stranding and fluid.

Teaching points

Groove pancreatitis is an uncommon form of focal chronic pancreatitis that involves the groove between the head of the pancreas, duodenum, and common bile duct. The adjacent pancreatic parenchyma can be spared as in the pure form, where it exclusively affects the groove, or involved segmentally in the process. The duodenum is always incorporated into the chronic inflammatory process. The pathogenesis is somewhat unclear but theories suggest pancreatic outflow obstruction via the duct of Santorini through the minor papilla. Other causes include cicatrisation in this anatomical space following acute pancreatitis in heterotopic pancreas. A pseudocyst can form due to cystic dystrophy of the heterotopic pancreas in the duodenal wall. It is commonly seen in alcoholics where Brunner gland hyperplasia causes obstruction at the minor ampulla. Groove pancreatitis is a sheet-like mass between the head of the pancreas and the C-loop of the duodenum. It is hypointense relative to the pancreas on T1-WI. It has variable appearance on T2-WI.

Management

Treatment is usually conservative. If surgery is required because of pain, a Whipple procedure or pylorus-sparing pancreaticoduodenectomy can be performed.

Further Readings

1. Castell-Monsalve F, Sousa-Martin J, Carazza A. Groove pancreatitis: MRI and pathological findings. *Abdominal Imaging.* 2008; *22*:342–348.
2. Blassbalg R, Baroni R, Costa D et al. MRI features of groove pancreatitis. *Am J Roentgenol.* 2007; *189*:73–80.

History

► 47-year-old man with chronic abdominal pain.

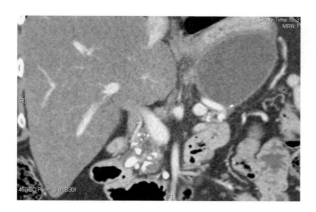

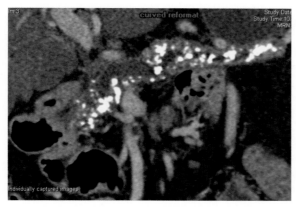

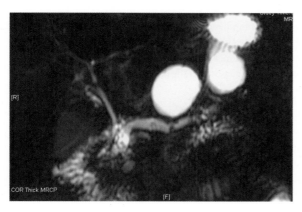

Case 135 Chronic Pancreatitis with Pseudocyst

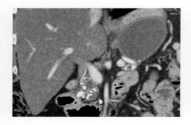 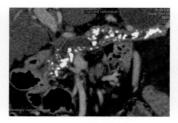 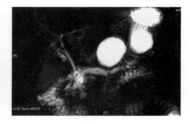

Findings

Contrast-enhanced coronal (left) CT image demonstrates coarse calcifications within the head image of the pancreas. A large pseudocyst is seen in the region of the tail of the pancreas. Coronal curved reformat image (middle) demonstrates pancreatic atrophy, coarse calcifications and main pancreatic duct dilatation with intraductal calcifications. Coronal thick slab MRCP image (right) in the same patient shows pancreatic duct dilatation with presence of two pseudocysts.

Differential Diagnosis

▶ Serous microcystic pancreatic adenoma: lobulated lesion, usually in head of pancreas, composed of multiple cysts measuring 0.2–2.0 cm. May have central stellate scar and calcification along the septae in a sunburst pattern.
▶ Mucinous cystic neoplasm: large cystic lesion with multiple enhancing septations, papillary projections and solid intramural nodules. Nearly exclusively seen in middle-aged females.
▶ Intraductal papillary mucinous neoplasm: cystic dilatation of the pancreatic duct and side branches due to epithelial production of mucin. Tends to be pleomorphic in shape and communication is seen with the main duct.
▶ SPT (solid pseudopapillary tumor of the pancreas): diagnosed in young female patients; may be a large purely cystic lesion or may be completely solid, may have hemorrhagic or necrotic internal architecture.

Teaching Points

Pseudocysts usually form approximately six weeks after an episode of acute pancreatitis, chronic pancreatitis, and secondary to trauma or surgery. They are localized amylase-rich fluid collections. Amylase values of less than 250 IU/ml virtually exclude a pseudocyst. They arise within or adjacent to pancreatic parenchyma and are surrounded by a thin smooth or uniform thick fibrous wall with no epithelial lining. They are usually unilocular but may indeed be multilocular and have internal debris. On CT, they usually are of fluid attenuation value. Post-contrast they may demonstrate enhancement of the wall. On MRI, they are predominantly hyperintense relative to pancreatic parenchyma on T2-weighted imaging and again may demonstrate wall enhancement post-contrast. Complications of pseudo include infection which has an associated high morbidity and mortality rate, hemorrhage, or rupture. Large pseudo can cause compression of adjacent pancreatic parenchyma and obstruct the downstream pancreatic duct or can cause pressure on adjacent intra-abdominal organs.

Management

Endoscopic ultrasound with or without fine needle aspiration can provide a specific diagnosis of pseudocyst in 69 percent and 85 percent of cases, respectively. Management is usually conservative if a pseudocyst measures less than 6 cm and is asymptomatic, because these often resolve spontaneously. If large or symptomatic or associated with infection, pseudocysts can be drained percutaneously or by endoscopic cyst-gastrostomy. In chronic cases, internal derivation and/or resection may be necessary.

Further Readings

1. Soliani P, Franzini C, Ziegler S, et al. Pancreatic pseudocysts following acute pancreatitis: risk factors influencing therapeutic outcomes. *J Pancreas*. 2004; 5(5): 338–347.
2. Young K, Saini S, Sahani D, et al. Imaging diagnosis of cystic pancreatic lesions: pseudocyst versus non-pseudocyst. *RadioGraphics*. 2005; 25:671–685.

History

▶ 68-year-old woman with early satiety and intermittent abdominal pain.

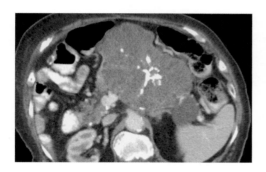

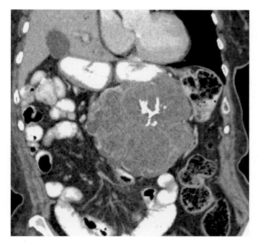

Case 136 Pancreatic Serous Cystadenoma (Microcystic Adenoma)

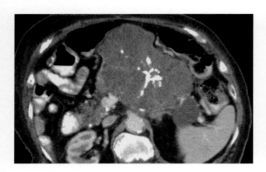 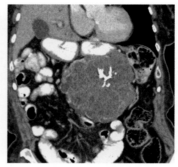

Findings

CT images show a large, well-circumscribed, solitary, lobulated multicystic mass within the pancreatic body. The mass contains innumerable small cysts and a central stellate calcified scar. There is no capsule, mural nodules, pancreatic duct irregularity, or parenchymal atrophy.

Differential Diagnosis

► Mucinous cystic neoplasm: usually occurs in middle-aged women and is located in the pancreatic body and tail. Common features include cysts larger than 2 cm, a definable capsule, oval or round shape, unilocular or few septations, and peripheral calcification. Enhancing soft tissue components suggest cystadenocarcinoma.

► Side branch intraductal papillary mucinous neoplasm: occurs in men and women. Establishing that the lesion is a dilated duct or communicates with the main pancreatic duct makes the diagnosis.

► Solid pseudopapillary tumor of the pancreas: rare encapsulated solid lesion occurring in young women. It appears cystic after hemorrhagic degeneration. It has no location predilection. Enhancing soft tissue component is uniformly present.

Teaching Points

Pancreatic serous cystadenoma is a rare benign cystic neoplasm of the pancreas that is most common in older women (mean age, 65 years). It is often referred to as microcystic adenoma and classically contains numerous cysts of various sizes (0.1 to 2.0 cm) that form a polycystic (70 percent) or honeycomb (20 percent) pattern. Ten percent of cases have an oligocystic or macrocystic pattern. Solid variants are exceedingly rare. Histologically, the cysts are lined by glycogen-rich epithelium. The septations coalesce into a central fibrous scar, which may calcify. Serous cystadenomas are almost exclusively solitary except in the setting of von Hippel-Lindau syndrome. Most lesions are incidentally discovered. Patients with large lesions may have pain and bloating.

Management

Imaging can make the diagnosis, and if the patient is asymptomatic, these lesions can safely be observed. If there is uncertainty regarding the diagnosis, characterization with endoscopic ultrasonography and fine needle aspiration is performed. Surgery may also be considered in a large or symptomatic lesion.

Further Reading

1. Hyoung JK, Ding HL, Young TK et al. CT of serous cystadenoma of the pancreas and Mimicking masses. *Am J Roentgenol.* 2008; *190*: 406–412.

History

▶ 55-year-old woman with left upper quadrant pain.

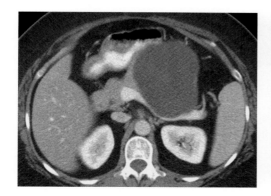
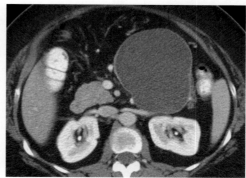
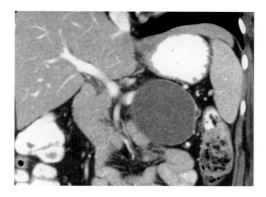

Case 137   Mucinous Cystic Neoplasm

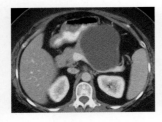 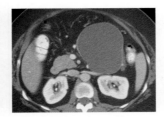 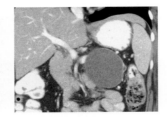

Findings

CT shows a well-circumscribed, encapsulated, low-attenuation mass in the body and tail of the pancreas. No pancreatic duct dilatation. The mass is solitary and no internal septa are seen.

Differential Diagnosis

► Intraductal papillary mucinous neoplasm (IPMN): a mucin-producing neoplasm that arises from the pancreatic duct and therefore communicates with the duct. IPMN is not encapsulated and is frequently pleomorphic in shape.
► Pseudocyst: also encapsulated but unlikely without history or findings of acute or chronic pancreatitis.
► Serous cystadenoma: most commonly has multiple cysts that are smaller than 2 cm. Serous tumors are not encapsulated.

Teaching Points

Mucinous cystic neoplasms of the pancreas are seen almost exclusively in women with a mean age at diagnosis of 53 years. They tend to occur in the body or tail of the pancreas. They present as solitary masses with single or multiple large cysts, each cyst measuring usually greater 2 cm. They may contain a solid component, such as mural nodules or papillary projections. Mucinous cystic neoplasm does not communicate with the pancreatic duct. Thin peripheral calcifications may be present in the septations or fibrous capsule bordering the tumor, but are seen in only 15 percent of cases. These tumors have malignant potential and therefore tend to be treated more aggressively than other pancreatic cystic lesions. The reported rate of invasive carcinoma ranges from 6 percent to 36 percent.

Management

Endoscopic ultrasound fine needle-aspiration of cyst contents can help to differentiate between serous cystadenomas, mucinous cystic neoplasm, and pseudocysts. Mucinous cystadenomas cannot be differentiated from cystadenocarcinomas based on imaging findings unless metastatic disease is present. Given the risk of malignancy, these are usually managed by surgical resection. Smaller lesions (less than 2 cm) can be treated with enucleation rather than pancreatic resection, given the low risk of malignancy in these lesions.

Further Reading

1. Parra-Herran CE, Garcia MT, et al. Cystic lesions of the pancreas: clinical and pathologic review of cases in a five-year period. *JOP: Journal of the pancreas.* 2010; *11*(4): 358–364.

History

► 28-year-old woman with an incidental pancreatic lesion.

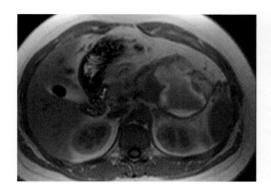
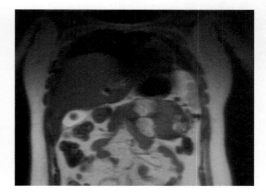
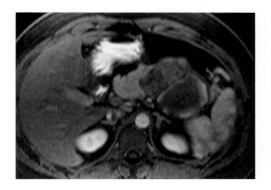

Case 138   Solid Pseudopapillary Tumor

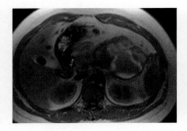 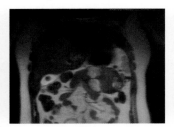 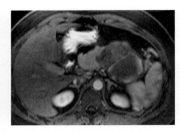

Findings

T1-, T2-images show a large, heterogenous, encapsulated mass in the tail of the pancreas. T1-weighted images show areas of high signal intensity consistent with hemorrhage. Post-contrast fat-saturated T1-weighted image confirm the presence of both cystic and solid components.

Differential Diagnosis

► Pseudocyst with complex fluid: encapsulated lesion with a clinical history or signs of acute or chronic pancreatitis.
► Mucinous cystic neoplasm: nearly exclusively located in the pancreatic body and tail and rarely has internal hemorrhage.
► Pancreatic endocrine tumor: may be cystic and encapsulated.

Teaching Points

Solid pseudopapillary tumors are low-grade malignancies of the pancreas occuring most often in young women (mean age, 25 to 27 years). Rare cases have been reported in males (male-to-female ratio is 1:9.5). Patients are frequently asymptomatic although they may have vague abdominal pain, poor appetite or nausea. Ultrasound or CT may show a well defined, encapsulated complex mass with both cystic and solid components. MRI is more sensitive than CT for detecting the cystic or solid components. Internal hemorrhage is very common. MRI is also more sensitive and specific than CT for detecting blood products within the lesion. If necessary, percutaneous or EUS guided aspiration can help differentiate this lesion from other cystic neoplasms of the pancreas. However, needle track seeding with tumor cells has been reported.

Management

Although the malignant potential of this tumor is low, radical resection is the treatment of choice, even in the presence of local recurrence or metastases. The choice of procedure depends on the location of the tumor. Local resection or enucleation can be performed for small tumors. Extensive lymphatic dissection is not recommended due to the low rate of lymph node involvement (3 percent). SPT is limited to the pancreas in 95 percent of patients and the local recurrence rate is less than 10 percent. Overall, the five-year survival is 95 percent.

Further Reading

1. Cantisani V, Mortele KJ et al. MR imaging features of solid pseudopapilary tumor of the pancreas in adult and pediatric patients. *Am J Roentgenol.*2003; *181*(2): 395–401.

History

▶ 71-year-old woman with weight loss and abdominal pain.

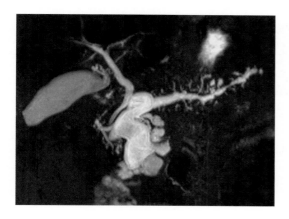

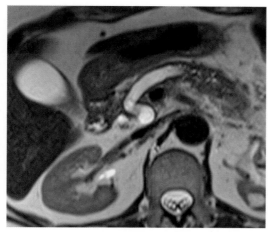

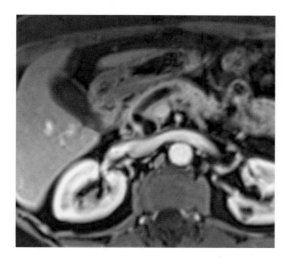

Case 139 Combined-Duct Type IPMN

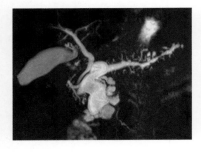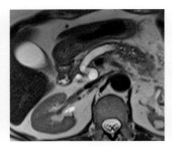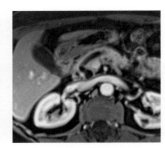

Findings

MRCP (left), T2-weighted (center), and portal venous phase post contrast T1-weighted (right) images show severe diffuse dilation of the main pancreatic duct throughout the entire pancreas. Associated dilatation of several side branches gives the pancreas a multicystic appearance but with no obstructing masses seen.

Differential Diagnosis

▶ Chronic pancreatitis: associated with focal or diffuse atrophy of the pancreas, with obstruction and dilatation of pancreatic/bile ducts and intraductal calculi, areas of calcification and stricturing, and chronic abdominal pain.

▶ Pancreatic pseudocyst: collection of pancreatic fluid encapsulated by fibrous capsule, not uncommonly associated with inflammatory changes in peripancreatic fat. MRCP may demonstrate communication of cystic lesion with main pancreatic duct. Clinical history of pancreatitis or alcoholism.

▶ Mucinous cystic neoplasm: round or oval, encapsulated, septated, and lobulated mass, commonly located in the pancreatic tail and with normal pancreatic duct. Multilocularity, mural nodules, thick wall, favor dysplasia or malignancy.

Teaching Points

Intraductal papillary mucinous neoplasm (IPMN) is a distinct clinicopathologic entity that is being recognized with increasing frequency. Typical features include a markedly dilated MPD with adjacent cystic lesions in the uncinate process and pancreatic head, representing mucin produced by the intraductal tumor, in the absence of an obstructing lesion. The tumor itself is rarely identified at imaging. A "gaping papilla" productive of mucin is a common finding on ERCP. There is communication between the cystic branches and the dilated ductal system.

Management

IPMNs have a low but well documented malignant progression rate. For this reason, an aggressive surgical approach is often recommended, with surgical resection of the entire potentially malignant lesion. This is particularly true in cases of main-duct and combined type IPMN, which carry a greater risk of underlying dysplasia or malignancy.

Further Reading

1. Prasad SR, Sahani D, Nasser S, et al. Intraductal papillary mucinous tumors of the pancreas. *Abdom Imaging.* 2003; 28:357–365.

History

▶ 66-year-old asymptomatic man.

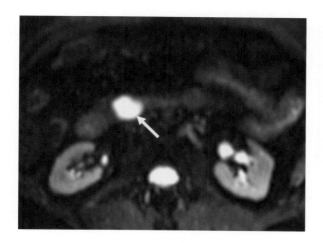

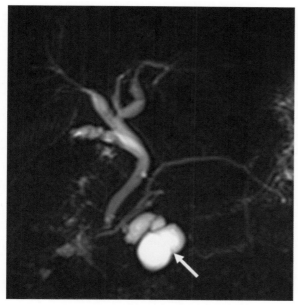

Case 140   Side Branch Intraductal Papillary Mucinous Neoplasm (IPMN)

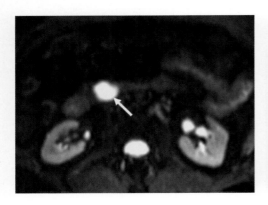 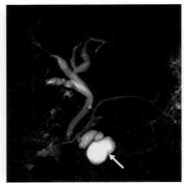

Findings

QWI (left) and thick slab MRCP (right) show a T2 hyperintense cyst in the uncinate process of the pancreatic head (white arrows). The mass communicates with a normal main pancreatic duct. There are no mural nodules.

Differential Diagnosis

► Mucinous cystic neoplasm: usually occurs in middle-aged women and is most commonly located in the distal pancreas. Common features include a definable capsule, oval or round shape, unilocular or few septations, and peripheral calcification. Enhancing soft tissue components suggest invasive cystadenocarcinoma.

► Pancreatic pseudocyst: occurs in patients with a history of pancreatitis. Background features of pancreatitis are usually present.

► Solid pseudopapillary tumor of the pancreas: rare lesions most commonly occurring in young women and have no location predilection. Enhancing soft tissue component is uniformly present and they do not communicate with the pancreatic duct. A capsule and internal hemorrhage are almost always present.

Teaching Points

Intraductal papillary mucinous neoplasm (IPMN) is a neoplasm that arises within the pancreatic duct. It can be subdivided into side branch, main duct, and combined type lesions. The main duct and combined type have a 60 percent to 70 percent likelihood of carcinoma, while approximately 15 percent of side branch lesions have foci of carcinoma. IPMNs are often multifocal and, in the case of side branch lesions, show communication with the main pancreatic duct. Side branch IPMNs are often asymptomatic and are incidentally discovered. On CT, IPMNs are hypoattenuating avascular lesions without a capsule or imaging evidence of chronic pancreatitis. Both CT and MRCP reliably detect cyst communication with the main pancreatic duct.

Management

Management of side branch IPMN remains a topic of much debate. Currently, asymptomatic patients with lesions measuring less than 3 cm may undergo follow-up imaging while patients with symptoms or lesions greater then 3 cm warrant fine needle aspiration along with surgical consultation for possible resection.

Further Reading

1. Song SJ, Lee JM, Kim YJ, et al. Differentiation of Intraductal Papillary Mucinous Neoplasms From Other Pancreatic Cystic Masses: Comparison of Multirow-detector CT and MR Imaging Using ROC Analysis. *J Magn Reson Imaging* 2007; *26*: 86–93.

History

▶ 50-year-old woman with hypoglycemia.

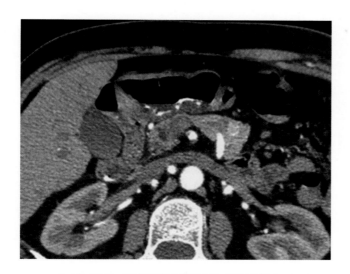

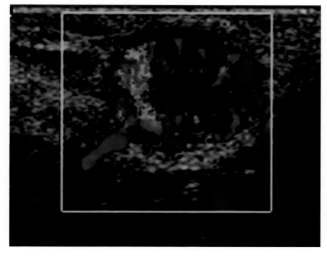

Case 141 Insulinoma

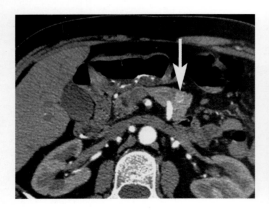 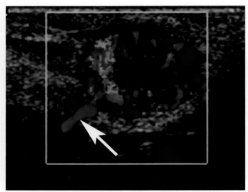

Findings

Axial CT image in the arterial phase (left) shows a small hypervascular mass (arrow) in the pancreatic body. Intraoperative pancreatic ultrasound (right) reveals prominent internal tumor vascularity and a visible feeding vessel (arrow) extending to the mass.

Differential Diagnosis

▶ Pancreatic adenocarcinoma: Hypovascular, infiltrative mass, usually with pancreatic ductal obstruction.
▶ Mucinous cystic tumor: Typically more of a unilocular cystic mass, but can appear similar to a cystic and/or necrotic islet cell tumor.

Teaching Points

Pancreatic endocrine tumors (a.k.a. neuroendocrine or islet cell tumors) arise from pancreatic islets, are usually solitary and sporadic, and are generally nonsyndromic and clinically silent. Syndromic or hyperfunctioning tumors are usually smaller sized and can be difficult to visualize. Pancreatic endocrine tumors are classified according to the predominant oversecreted hormone, and insulinomas account for about half of pancreatic endocrine tumors. Clinically, patients with a hyperfunctioning insulinoma present with hypoglycemia and have continued secretion of insulin despite a lower glucose level and relief of symptoms with IV glucose (Whipple triad). The majority of insulinomas are benign, solitary, and less than 2 cm. At CT, the typical appearance is a well circumscribed, hypervascular mass, best seen on arterial phase. There is usually no duct obstruction, unlike pancreatic adenocarcinoma. Calcification is present in up to 20 percent of cases. On ultrasound, the mass is often hypoechoic and well circumscribed with increased vascularity. Intraoperative ultrasound is helpful to localize small tumors and delineate the tumors' relationship to the main pancreatic duct and adjacent vessels. Tumors can be subtle on imaging. Metastatic lesions, mostly in the liver, are hypervascular similar to the primary tumor. Regional adenopathy, and liver, bone and pulmonary metastases can be seen.

Management

Resection is the only definitive curative treatment, so local staging is critical. Intraoperative ultrasonography helps identify additional tumors. Chemotherapy, interferon and octreotide, hepatic artery embolization or ligation may also be attempted.

Further Reading

1. Rappeport ED, Hansen CP, Kjaer A, Knigge U. Multidetector computed tomography and neuroendocrine pancreaticoduodenal tumors. *Acta Radiol*. 2006 Apr; 47(3):248–56.

History

▶ 65-year-old woman with right upper quadrant pain and weight loss.

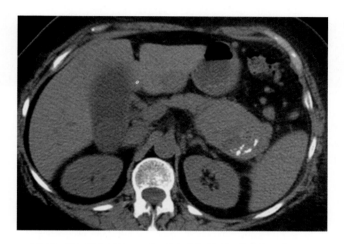

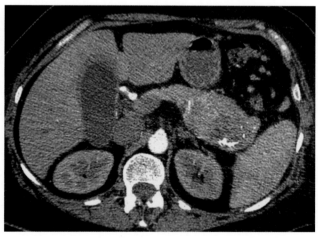

Case 142 Non-Hyperfunctioning Pancreatic Endocrine Tumor

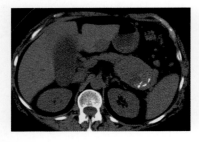 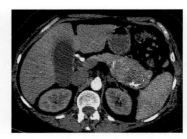 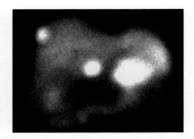

Findings

CT scan (left) shows a large mass in the tail of the pancreas that contains coarse calcifications and enhances with intravenous contrast. There are areas of hypoattenuating necrosis (middle). The gallbladder is distended and has wall thickening. Complementary octreotide scintigraphy (right) shows uptake in the pancreatic mass and liver metastasis.

Differential Diagnosis

► Pancreatic adenocarcinoma: may present similarly as a large mass in the tail of the pancreas and metastatic lesions in the liver. Pancreatic adenocarcinomas do not typically have calcifications, are ill-defined, and are not active on octreotide scintigraphy.

► Hyperfunctioning endocrine tumor of the pancreas: diagnosis is made biochemically when patients present with symptoms related to a specific hormonal syndrome. As such, functional tumors are more likely to be recognized when tumors are small.

► Metastatic disease: metastatic lesions, such as from renal cell carcinoma, colon cancer, and melanoma, may appear similar to pancreatic endocrine tumors and other primary pancreatic neoplasms.

Teaching Points

Pancreatic endocrine tumors arise from the pancreatic endocrine cells. Fifteen to thirty percent of pancreatic endocrine tumors are classified as non-hyperfunctioning. Tumors are characterized as non-hyperfunctioning if the secreted tumor substance does not cause specific symptoms. CT is commonly utilized to localize and stage pancreatic endocrine tumors. These are more common in the tail of the pancreas compared to adenocarcinoma, and are more likely to have areas of necrosis, hemorrhage, and calcification. These soft tumors generally do not cause substantial pancreatic duct dilatation. Non-hyperfunctioning tumors are generally larger at the time of diagnosis compared to hyperfunctioning tumors because they do not produce clinical symptoms in the early stages of disease. Patients may complain of nonspecific symptoms, including weight loss, abdominal pain, jaundice, fatigue, and abdominal distention. Approximately 60 to 90 percent of non-hyperfunctioning tumors have malignant biologic behavior.

Management

Octreotide scintigraphy is useful for staging and preoperative planning because it is more sensitive for the detection of small lymph node and liver metastasis compared to CT. Surgical resection is the only treatment with the potential for cure.

Further Reading

1. Rockall AG and Reznek RH. Imaging of neuroendocrine tumours (CT/MR/US). *Best Practice & Research Clinical Endocrinology & Metabolism.* 2007; 21:43–68.

History

▶ 37-year-old man with epigastric pain.

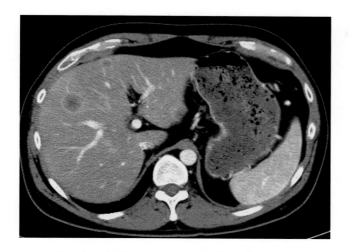

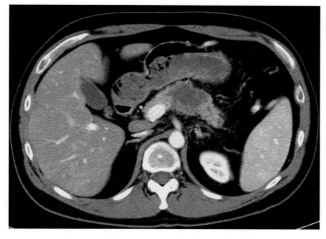

Case 143 Pancreatic Adenocarcinoma

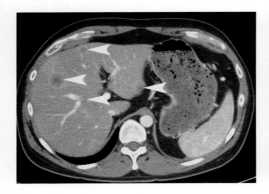 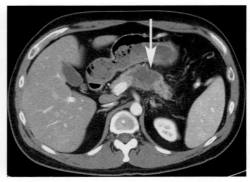

Findings

Axial contrast-enhanced CT shows a large, irregular heterogeneous hypoenhancing mass in the body of the pancreas (arrow) with atrophy of the tail of the pancreas and a dilated upstream pancreatic duct. Round hypoattenuating metastases (arrowheads) are seen in the liver.

Differential Diagnosis

▶ Endocrine tumor: typically show hyperenhancement in the arterial phase and tend not to cause pancreatic duct dilatation. May have symptoms related to hormone production.

▶ Chronic pancreatitis: intraductal calculi and parenchymal calcification are often present, which is uncommon for pancreatic adenocarcinoma.

Teaching Points

Most (85 to 95 percent) pancreatic cancers are adenocarcinomas. These cancers have poor prognosis, with 1-year survival of less than 20 percent, dropping to under 5 percent by 5 years. Although typically hypodense, approximately 10 percent of adenocarcinomas are isodense to pancreatic parenchyma; their presence must be inferred from contour abnormality, duct obstruction, or vascular invasion. Pancreatic adenocarcinoma is curable only by resection, but most cases are unresectable at time of diagnosis. Failed attempts at surgical resection lead to substantial patient morbidity. Therefore, it is critical to identify unresectable tumor at CT and MR staging. Findings that make complete resection improbable include vascular involvement, tumor size greater than 4 cm, and distant metastases. Vascular involvement is suggested when veins are narrowed by tumor or when tumor contacts more than a 180-degree circumference of a blood vessel, and the most common vessels to be involved are the superior mesenteric and celiac vessels. Multiplanar images are helpful in establishing these findings. The most common sites of metastasis are the liver and peritoneum.

Management

The main purpose of imaging is to exclude unresectable tumor and to identify urgent findings that require palliative treatment, such as bowel or bile duct obstruction.

Further Reading

1. Low G, Panu A, Millo N, Leen E. Multimodality imaging of neoplastic and nonneoplastic solid lesions of the pancreas. *RadioGraphics.* 2011; *31*:993–1015.

History

▶ 65-year-old man with a prior left nephrectomy for renal cell carcinoma.

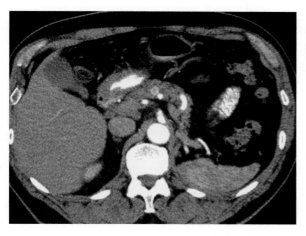

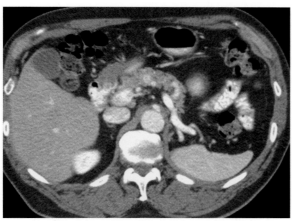

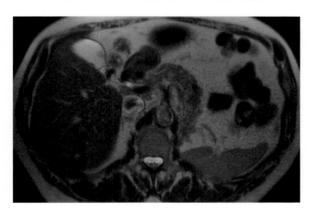

Case 144 Pancreatic Metastasis from Renal Cell Carcinoma

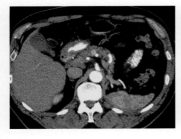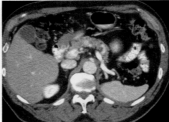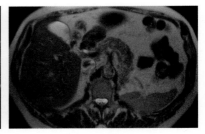

Findings

CT images obtained during the arterial phase (left) and a portal venous phase (middle) of contrast enhancement show an 8 mm hyperenhancing lesion in the body of the pancreas. T2-weighted MR image shows a heterogeneously hyperintense well circumscribed mass.

Differential Diagnosis

▶ Endocrine tumor of the pancreas: may have an identical appearance to highly vascular metastasis.
▶ Serous cystadenoma: has a lobulated contour and typically contains numerous small cysts with a central scar.
▶ Solid pseudopapillary tumor: encapsulated and most often occurs in young women.

Teaching Points

The most common primary tumor producing pancreatic metastases is renal cell carcinoma, followed by lung, breast, sarcoma, colon cancer, and melanoma. Rare case reports have been published of pancreatic metastases from uterine cancer, choriocarcinoma, and liposarcoma. Compared to pancreatic adenocarcinoma, which is usually hypoenhancing compared to pancreatic parenchyma, metastases tend to demonstrate either peripheral hyperenhancement (more than 70 percent) or homogeneous enhancement. Thus, the main differential for these lesions is endocrine tumor of the pancreas. Three patterns of involvement are recognized: solitary (50 to 70 percent), diffuse (15 to 44 percent), and multifocal (5 to 10 percent). The presence of additional intra-abdominal metastases or a known malignancy can be helpful in making the diagnosis.

Management

Pancreatic metastases are rare. Most patients with pancreatic metastases have widespread disease at the time of detection and as such are not candidates for resection. Small case series have described encouraging results with resection for isolated pancreatic metastases from RCC. Locally directed treatments, such as cyberknife radiosurgery, have had some success. However, long-term results are not yet available.

Further Reading

1. Low G, Panu A, et al. Multimodality imaging of neoplastic and nonneoplastic solid lesions of the pancreas. *RadioGraphics*. 2011; *31*(4):993–1015.

History

▶ 45-year-old man with headache and abdominal pain.

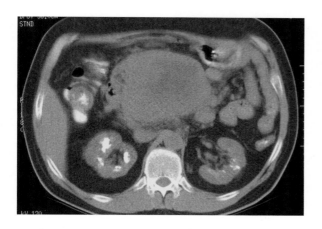

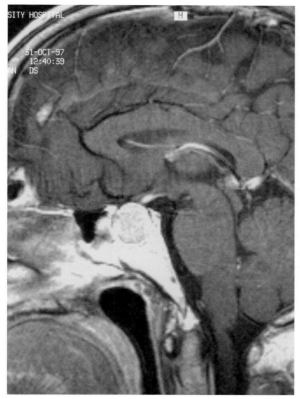

Case 145   Multiple Endocrine Neoplasia Type 1

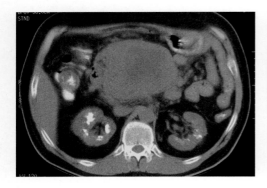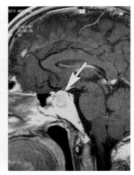

Findings

Enhanced CT through the level of the pancreas shows a large heterogeneous mass in the body of the pancreas. Bilateral renal medullary calcification is present. Sagittal gadolinium-enhanced T1-weighted MRI of the brain shows an enhancing pituitary mass (arrow).

Differential Diagnosis

► The combination of a pituitary mass typical of an adenoma, pancreatic mass, and medullary nephrocalcinosis is pathognomonic for MEN-1 syndrome.

Teaching Points

Multiple endocrine neoplasia type 1 (MEN-1), also known as Werner syndrome, is an autosomal dominant condition, characterized by parathyroid adenomas, pancreatic endocrine tumors, and anterior pituitary adenomas. Patients may also develop gastrin-secreting carcinoids of the duodenum, thymic, and bronchial carcinoids, and pheochromocytomas. The renal medullary calcification and recurrent renal stones in MEN-1 are due to hyperparathyroidism, which may be secondary to parathyroid adenomas or parathyroid hyperplasia, and occur in 88 to 97 percent of MEN-1 patients. Noninvasive imaging tests, including nuclear medicine scintigraphy and ultrasound, have a high sensitivity for localizing parathyroid disease, and may be needed for parathyroid localization. Patients have elevated serum calcium and elevated parathyroid hormone levels. Functional and nonfunctional endocrine tumors of the pancreas are reported to occur in 30 to 80 percent of patients with MEN-1. Malignant progression of these tumors is a principle cause of mortality in patients with MEN-1. Gastrinomas are the most common functional endocrine tumors in patients with MEN-1, followed by insulinomas. Gastrinomas may also occur in the duodenum or paraduodenal tissues within the gastrinoma triangle. CT is commonly the imaging modality used for localization of these tumors. Patients with hypergastrinemia may develop Zollinger-Ellison syndrome. Anterior pituitary adenomas occur in 15 to 80 percent of MEN-1 patients. These tumors are usually functional and secrete prolactin (most commonly) or growth hormone (second most common). Pituitary macroadenomas may cause symptoms by compressing on adjacent structures.

Management

MEN-1 is a multisystem disorder that can be managed, but not cured. A combination of medical, surgical and oncologic treatments is often necessary for these patients.

Further Reading

1. Scarsbrook AF, Thakker RV, Wass JA, Gleeson FV, Phillips RR. Multiple endocrine neoplasia: spectrum of radiologic appearances and discussion of a multitechnique imaging approach. *RadioGraphics*. 2006; 26(2):433–451.

History

► 35-year-old woman with incidental pancreatic mass identified in the tail during abdominal CT performed to evaluate abdominal pain.

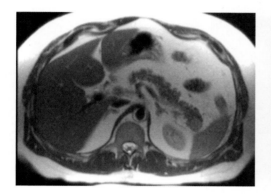 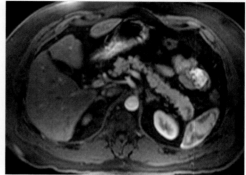

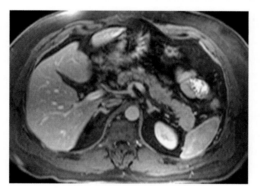

Case 146 Intrapancreatic Accessory Spleen

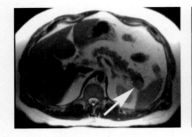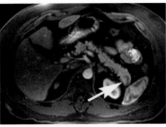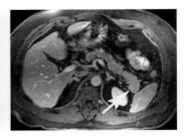

Findings

Axial T2-weighted (left), post contrast FS T1-weighted in the arterial phase (middle) and portal venous phase (right) show a round lesion (arrows) in the tail of the pancreas that is isointense to the spleen on all pulse sequences.

Differential Diagnosis

► Splenosis nodule: usually the result of trauma, caused by implantation of portions of the disrupted spleen anywhere, including abdomen, pelvis, and chest. The implanted tissue continues to function and may occasionally enlarge.
► Pancreatic endocrine tumor: tumors arising from pancreatic endocrine cells (islets of Langerhans), consisting of hyperfunctioning and nonhyperfunctioning tumors. They are usually hypervascular, often demonstrating internal necrosis and cystic areas. The presence of calcifications is not uncommon.

Teaching Points

Ectopic splenic tissue can be separated into two categories: splenosis due to autotransplanation of splenic tissue, which usually occurs after splenectomy, and accessory spleens, which are congenital foci of splenic tissue in an ectopic location, usually in the left upper quadrant, above the renal pedicle. In rare cases, it may be embedded within the pancreatic tail, as demonstrated in this case. Ectopic splenic tissue should always be suspected in the context of a small nodule (less than 2.5 cm) with the same signal characteristics and enhancement pattern as normal spleen.

Management

Differentiating ectopic splenic tissue from other pancreatic masses is extremely important and can spare patients unnecessary surgical treatment. The diagnosis can be made with the combination of the characteristic location of the lesion along with signal intensities that were identical to the spleen on multiple pulse sequences. Confirmation of accessory spleen in the pancreas can be obtained with scintigraphy; technetium-labeled sulfur colloid or heat-damaged RBC offers functional or physiologic images and is therefore highly specific for differentiating spleen from other tissues. Treatment is conservative if imaging features are consistent with accessory spleen and if the patient is asymptomatic. In rare cases of hypersplenism or recurrence of lymphoma, surgical resection is indicated.

Further Readings

1. Sahni VA, Mortelé KJ. The Bloody Pancreas: MDCT and MRI Features of Hypervascular and Hemorrhagic Pancreatic Conditions. *Am J Roentgenol.* 2009; *192*:923–935.
2. Mortele KJ, Mortele B, Silverman SG. CT Features of the Accessory Spleen. *Am J Roentgenol.* 2004; *183*:1653–1657.

History

► 56-year-old woman undergoing abdominal CT surveillance for metastases from an extremity sarcoma resected three years prior.

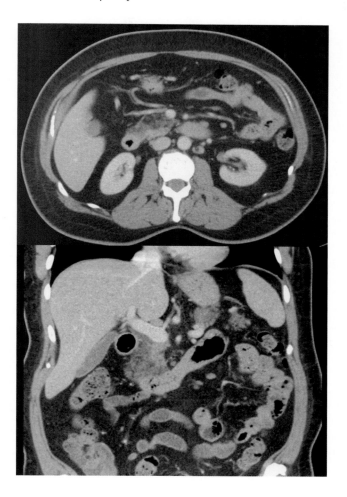

Case 147 Focal Fatty Change of the Pancreas

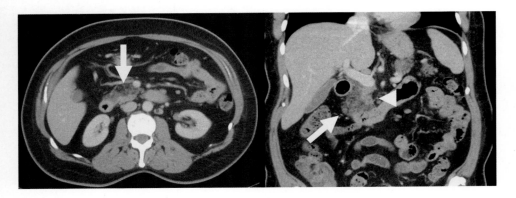

Findings

Axial (left) and coronal (right) CT images obtained during the portal venous phase of intravenous contrast enhancement depict non-mass-like fat deposition (arrow) admixed with slivers of normal pancreatic parenchyma in the pancreatic head. The fatty change spares the ventral anlage (arrowhead). The glandular margins are preserved. Pancreaticobiliary duct dilatation is absent.

Differential Diagnosis

▶ Pancreatic ductal adenocarcinoma: the desmoplastic response elicited by the tumor may present as a low-attenuation mass. However, there will typically be biliary and/or pancreatic duct obstruction as well as perivascular soft tissue infiltration.

▶ Retroperitoneal liposarcoma: pancreatic involvement by this tumor is rare and associated with mass-like expansion of regional fat that displaces adjacent structures.

▶ Pancreatic lipoma: focal, well defined island of fat surrounded by normal pancreas.

Teaching Points

Pancreatic lipomatosis may be focal or diffuse. Fatty replacement of the anterior pancreatic head (dorsal anlage) is the most common type of uneven pancreatic lipomatosis. The cause of this commonly seen fatty change is unclear, but appears to involve differences in the histological composition between the dorsal and ventral anlages and is a benign finding. Diffuse pancreatic lipomatosis may develop in elderly, diabetic, obese, cystic fibrosis, and Shwachman-Diamond syndrome patients.

Management

Focal pancreatic fatty change in the pancreas is of no clinical consequence unless it is misinterpreted as pathologic by the radiologist. If the diagnosis is questionable on CT, MR imaging using in/opposed phase T1-weighted sequences should demonstrate the presence of fat in the involved portion of the gland.

Further Readings

1. Mortelé KJ, Rocha TC, Streeter JL, et al. Multimodality imaging of pancreatic and biliary congenital anomalies. *RadioGraphics*. 2006; *26*:715–773.
2. Keppke AL, Miller FH. Magnetic resonance imaging of the pancreas: the future is now. *Semin Ultrasound CT MR*. 2005; *26*:132–152.

History

► 36-year-old woman with chronic abdominal pain.

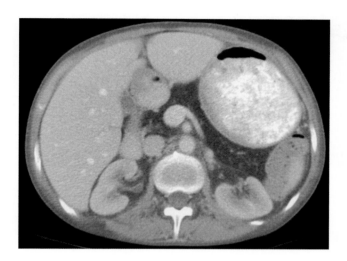

Case 148 Diffuse Fatty Replacement of the Pancreas Due to Cystic Fibrosis

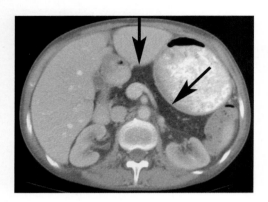

Findings

Contrast-enhanced CT images through the level of the pancreas show diffuse fatty replacement of the pancreatic parenchyma (arrows). No focal masses or adjacent inflammatory change are seen.

Differential Diagnosis

- ► Chronic pancreatitis: usually the pancreatic duct is irregularly dilated and some pancreatic parenchyma is still visible.
- ► Shwachman-Diamond syndrome: rare multisystem entity with profound pancreatic lipomatosis. Bronchiectasis, intestinal obstruction, or hepatic fibrosis are suggestive of cystic fibrosis.
- ► Insulin dependent diabetes mellitus: patient history is a useful discriminator.
- ► Nonspecific fatty atrophy: profuse fat with glandular atrophy may occur in the elderly, obese, or patients on chronic steroid therapy.

Teaching Points

Cystic fibrosis is an autosomal recessive disorder characterized by abnormalities of exocrine gland function. Pulmonary changes such as bronchiectasis, emphysema and sub-pleural blebs are the most frequent manifestations and the most common cause of morbidity and mortality. As management of pulmonary disease in this patient population continues to improve, life expectancy is increasing and abnormalities of other organs are increasingly recognized on imaging, particularly in adolescents and adults. Pancreatic abnormalities on imaging may be present in up to 85 to 90 percent of adolescent patients with cystic fibrosis and appears to increase with age. The etiology of pancreatic fatty replacement in cystic fibrosis is not well understood, and was once hypothesized as being due to thick secretions that cause progressive pancreatic atrophy and fibrosis with eventual fatty replacement. Arguments against this theory include the fact that patients with fatty pancreatic replacement rarely have dilated pancreatic ducts or a stronger association with pancreatic dysfunction than those without fatty replacement.

Management

Symptomatic patients are managed with dietary alterations and pancreatic enzyme replacement.

Further Reading

1. Soyer P, Spelle L, Pelage JP, Dufresne AC, et al. Cystic Fibrosis in Adolescents and Adults: Fatty Replacement of the Pancreas—CT Evaluation and Functional Correlation. *Radiology*. 1999; *210*:611–615.

History

▶ 24-year-old man with two-month history of abdominal pain.

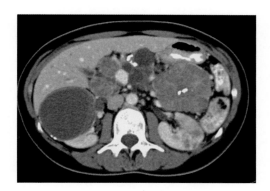

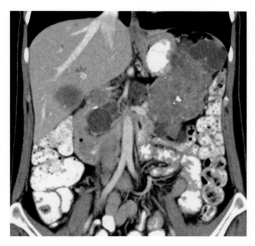

Case 149 Von Hippel Lindau Syndrome

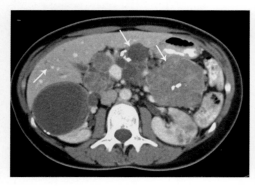
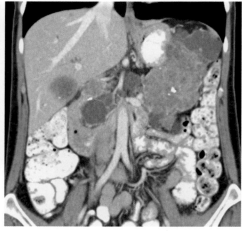

Findings

CT images show diffuse cystic replacement of the pancreas and multiple well-circumscribed, lobulated septated cysts in the pancreatic tail (arrows). The largest cystic mass in the pancreatic tail has central calcification. A complex thick-walled right renal cyst is present. It has enhancing septations as well as peripheral coarse calcification.

Differential Diagnosis

► Cystic fibrosis: complete fatty replacement is the most common pancreatic finding in adult patients. Pancreatic cysts are also relatively common. They are usually small, measuring 1–3 mm and are best shown with T2-weighted MR imaging. Occasionally, aggregates of true epithelium-lined cysts completely replace the pancreas, a condition referred to as pancreatic cystosis.

► Multiple IPMN: IPMNs are often multifocal and in the case of side branch lesions, demonstrate communication with the main pancreatic duct.

► Autosomal dominant polycystic kidney (hepatorenal) disease: renal cysts are present in one-half of patients by the age of 10 years. Pancreatic cysts occur in 10 percent of patients and are always associated with renal cysts. Pancreatic cystosis is not a feature of autosomal dominant polycystic kidney disease.

Teaching Points

Von Hippel-Lindau (VHL) is autosomal dominant with variable penetrance. It is characterized by retinal angiomas and central nervous system hemangioblastomas. Pancreatic cysts are common in VHL (50 to 91 percent). Pancreatic cysts range from a single cyst to cystic replacement of the entire gland. Peripheral calcification in the cyst wall may be present. Pancreatic neoplasms are also common in VHL (0 to 77 percent). They include serous cystadenomas (12 percent), endocrine tumors (5 to 15 percent), and rarely adenocarcinomas. Renal lesions (59 to 63 percent) also occur and may be solid or complex cystic renal cell carcinomas (24 to 45 percent), which are often bilateral. Pheochromocytomas and papillary cystadenomas of the epididymis also occur in these patients.

Management

Annual screening of the pancreas and kidneys with either ultrasound or CT is recommended in patients with VHL. Annual 24-hour measurement of urine vanillylmandelic acid (VMA) for pheochromocytoma is also recommended.

Further Reading

1. Leung RS, Biswas SV, Duncan M, et al. Imaging of von Hippel-Landau Disease. *RadioGraphics*. 2008; 28:65–79.

History

▶ 33-year-old man with history of alcoholism presenting with epigastric pain and high lipase and amylase levels. CT scan was performed seven days after hospital admission.

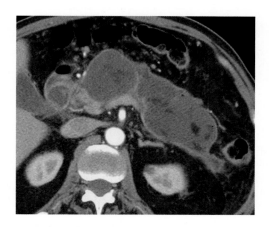

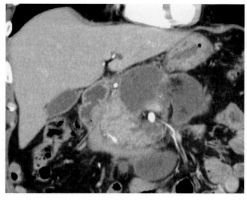

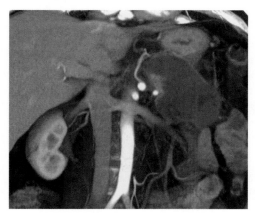

Case 150 Acute Necrotizing Pancreatitis

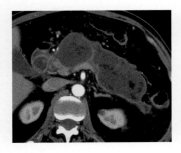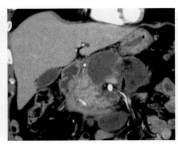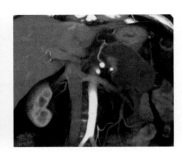

Findings

Axial (left) and coronal (center) contrast-enhanced CT images obtained in the late arterial (pancreatic) phase demonstrate extensive heterogeneous areas of nonenhancement involving predominantly the pancreatic body and tail, indicating pancreatic necrosis. A coronal volume-rendering technique 3D image (right) demonstrates the close relationship of the pancreatic necrosis with the surrounding structures, including the gastric body.

Differential Diagnosis

▶ Infiltrating pancreatic carcinoma: ill-defined, heterogeneous, poorly enhancing (hypovascular) mass, causing abrupt obstruction and dilatation of the pancreatic duct and obliteration of the retropancreatic fat. Weight loss and abdominal pain are not unusual clinical findings, although incidental detection has become increasingly more common.

▶ Lymphoma and metastases: nodular, or diffuse enlargement of the pancreatic parenchyma, commonly associated with retroperitoneal adenopathy.

Teaching Points

Acute inflammatory process of the pancreatic parenchyma, associated with variable involvement of other regional tissues and/or remote organ systems. Typical findings include enlargement of the pancreas, peripancreatic fat stranding and adjacent fluid collections. After contrast administration, heterogeneous enhancement is not uncommon, with nonenhancing areas corresponding to areas of necrosis. Common etiologies include alcohol, gallstones, infection, trauma, and drugs.

Management

In cases of noncomplicated (edematous) acute pancreatitis, treatment is usually conservative and basically supportive. However, the presence of necrosis is the most important prognostic imaging finding and is associated with higher incidence of complications, such as superimposed infection and multi-system organ failure. In cases of complicated pancreatitis, surgical, percutaneous, and/or endoscopic intervention is often needed. Given close proximity, an endoscopic transgastric approach is commonly used when drainage is indicated.

Further Readings

1. Balthazar EJ. Acute Pancreatitis: Assessment of Severity with Clinical and CT Evaluation. *Radiology.* 2002; *223*:603–613.
2. Mortele KJ, Wiesner W, Intriere L, et al. A Modified CT Severity Index for Evaluating Acute Pancreatitis: Improved Correlation with Patient Outcome. *Am J Roentgenol.* 2004; *183*:1261–1265.

Part 11   Spleen

History

▶ 13-year-old boy with acute lymphoblastic leukemia.

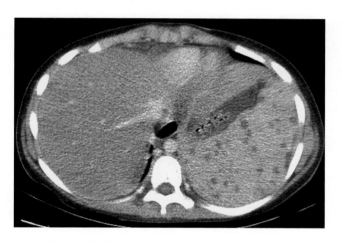

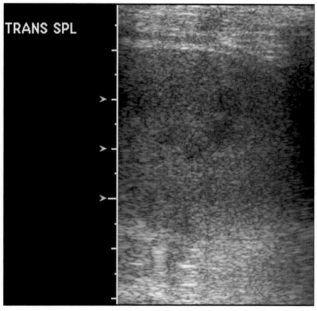

Case 151 Splenic Candidiasis

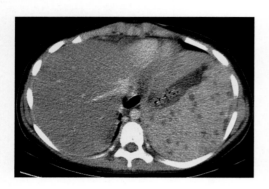

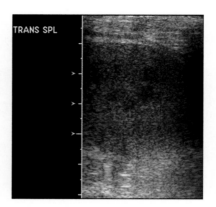

Findings

Axial contrast-enhanced CT of the spleen (left image) demonstrates multiple scattered small well-defined, round, non-enhancing, low-attenuation foci. In an immunocompromised patient, these are most compatible with microabscesses. These same lesions are hypoechoic (but not anechoic) on ultrasound (right image).

Differential Diagnosis

► Splenic metastases: variable imaging appearance. In particular, melanoma, ovarian, breast, and endometrial cancers can produce homogeneous hypoattenuating splenic metastases. Clinical setting helps with differentiation.

► Pyogenic abscess: typically larger in size and smaller in number or solitary. Borders are well defined but irregular. Rim enhancement may be seen.

► Leukemia deposits: may look identical to fungal micro-abscesses on imaging and may need fine needle aspiration for final differentiation. Shows rapid regression after cytostatic treatment.

Teaching Points

Splenic fungal infections occur almost exclusively in immunocompromised patients. The most common pathogen is *Candida*, followed by *Aspergillus* and *Cryptococcus*. Candidal infections often have the appearance seen in this case. When the lesions are larger, they may have concentric zones of higher and lower attenuation, a finding that has been referred to as "wheel within wheel." Rim enhancement is uncommon. Microabscesses may be too small to detect with imaging, so absence of these findings does not exclude the diagnosis.

Management

Historically, splenic fungal infections were treated with splenectomy. Recently, treatment with systemic antifungal medications has become more common as more effective medications have become available.

Further Readings

1. Chew FS, Smith PL, and Barboriak D. 1991. Candidal splenic abscesses. *Am J Roentgenol.* 1991. *156*: 474.
2. Freeman JL, Jafri SZ, Roberts JL, Mezwa DG, and Shirkhoda A. CT of congenital and acquired abnormalities of the spleen. *RadioGraphics.* 1993; *13*: 597–610.
3. Rabushka LS, Kawashima A, and Fishman EK. Imaging of the spleen: CT with supplemental MR examination. *RadioGraphics.* 1994; *14*: 307–332.

History

▶ 36-year-old man with multiple indeterminate splenic masses identified on CT scan performed to evaluate diffuse abdominal pain. MR imaging is performed to further characterize the splenic lesions.

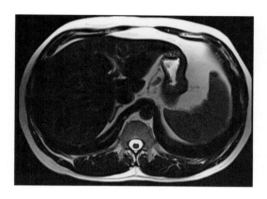

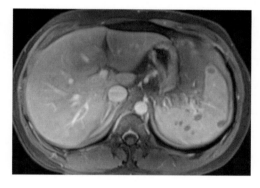

Case 152 Splenic Sarcoidosis

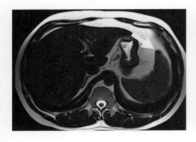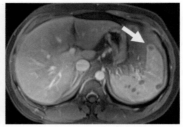

Findings

Axial T2-weighted MR image (left) demonstrates multiple rounded hypointense splenic masses (arrow) that are hypovascular to normal spleen on the axial contrast-enhanced fat-suppressed T1-weighted MR image obtained during portal venous phase (right). The spleen is not enlarged. No hepatic masses or lymphadenopathy are present.

Differential Diagnosis

▶ Lymphoma: often indistinguishable from sarcoidosis on imaging: may have associated regional lymphadenopathy and splenomegaly with or without multiple hypovascular and hypointense T1- and T2-weighted splenic masses.

▶ Littoral cell angioma: another cause of multiple hypovascular splenic masses of low T1 and T2 signal intensity. Patients typically exhibit splenomegaly and anemia or thrombocytopenia.

▶ Opportunistic fungal infection: fungal splenic microabscesses are generally seen in immunocompromised patients and may be indistinguishable from sarcoidosis by imaging alone. Liver involvement is typically present.

Teaching Points

Sarcoidosis is a systemic granulomatous disease of unknown etiology that may involve the spleen. Splenic involvement typically manifests as splenomegaly with or without numerous parenchymal nodules, which are hypovascular and hypointense on T1- and T2-weighted MR images relative to normal parenchyma, and may be occult on unenhanced CT scan. These nodules are the result of confluent noncaseating granulomas that can be seen in the absence of splenomegaly or abdominal lymphadenopathy. Hepatic nodules will be seen in approximately one-half of patients with splenic nodules. Approximately one-quarter of patients with sarcoidosis and splenic nodules will have no findings of sarcoidosis on chest radiographs.

Management

Patients with splenic involvement of sarcoidosis are often asymptomatic and frequently have elevated angiotensin converting enzyme (ACE) levels. While imaging may suggest the diagnosis of splenic sarcoidosis, biopsy or splenectomy may be required to exclude alternate diagnoses.

Further Readings

1. Warshauer DM. Splenic sarcoidosis. *Seminars in Ultrasound, CT and MRI*. 2007; *28*(1):21–27.
2. Kamaya A, Weinstein S, Desser TS. Multiple lesions of the spleen: differential diagnosis of cystic and solid lesions. *Seminars in Ultrasound, CT and MRI*. 2007; *28*(1):389–403.
3. Abbott RM, Levy AD, Aguilera NS, et al. From the archives of the AFIP: primary vascular neoplasms of the spleen: radio-logic-pathologic correlation. *RadioGraphics*. 2004; *24*:1137–1163.

History

► 36-year-old woman with acute shortness of breath and chest pain.

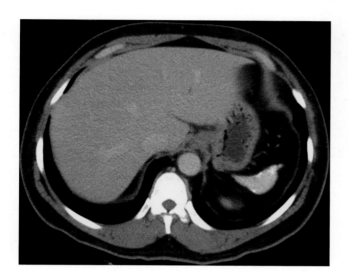

Case 153 Sickle Cell Disease with Splenic Autoinfarction

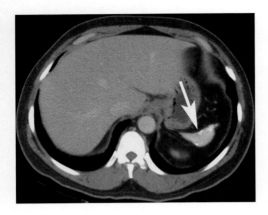

Findings

Contrast-enhanced CT image shows a shrunken and partially calcified spleen (arrow).

Differential Diagnosis

► Remote granulomatous disease: typically the size of the spleen will be preserved and will show punctate calcified granulomas in the spleen.

► Splenic siderosis: the spleen is of normal size but may appear diffusely dense due to iron deposition, frequently related to multiple prior blood transfusions.

Teaching Points

Sickle cell anemia is the most common genetic disorder affecting African Americans with a prevalence of 1 in 375, and a heterozygous gene carrier rate of 1 in 12. Sickle cell anemia is a hemolytic anemia characterized by abnormally shaped ("sickled") red blood cells, which are destroyed at increased rates, leading to anemia. Of greater clinical importance, the sickled red blood cells cause vascular occlusion, which leads to tissue ischemia and infarction. Many organ systems throughout the body are affected. leading to characteristic findings on imaging. The spleen is particularly susceptible to ischemia/infarction due to its slow microcirculation, and over time this results in autosplenectomy. Current data show that at the age of 2 years 58 percent of sickle cell anemia patients are functionally asplenic, with an increase to 94 percent of patients by 5 years of age. On radiographs or CT the spleen in patients with sickle cell anemia can appear small in size, dense, and calcified. MRI typically shows loss of signal in the splenic parenchyma on both T1 and T2 imaging due to fibrosis and ferrocalcinosis.

Management

Patients with functional asplenia are prone to encapsulated bacterial infections, specifically *S. Pneumoniae, H. Influenza, Salmonella*, and *Klebsiella*. Vaccination and oral antibiotic prophylaxis at an early age may reduce infection rates.

Further Readings

1. Lonergan GJ, Cline DB, Abbondanzo SL. Sickle Cell Disease. *RadioGraphics*. 2001; *21*:971–994.
2. Lane, PA. Sickle Cell Disease. *Pediatric Clin North Amer.* 1996; 43:639–664.

History

▶ 47-year-old woman undergoing abdominal MRI to evaluate incidentally detected splenic lesions.

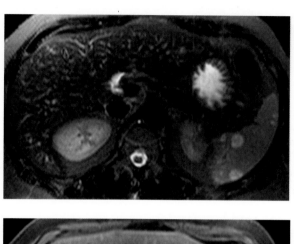

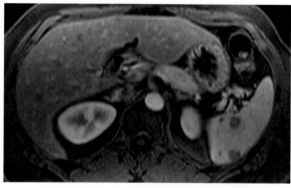

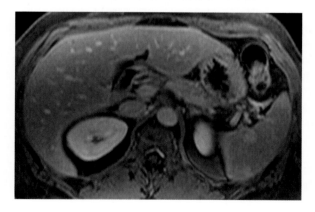

Case 154 Splenic Hemangiomata

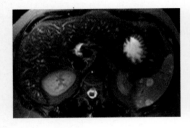 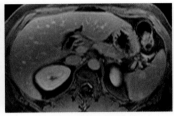 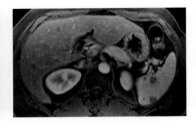

Findings

Axial fat-suppressed T2-weighted image demonstrates multiple well-circumscribed T2 hyperintense lesions in the spleen (left). These were mildly hypointense on pre-contrast T1-weighted images (not shown), and following intravenous gadolinium administration these lesions demonstrate early mottled enhancement (middle) with delayed hyperenhancement compared to the background spleen (right).

Differential Diagnosis

▶ Splenic cyst: hypoechoic on ultrasound, hypodense on CT and non-enhancing.
▶ Splenic hamartoma: typically isointense on T1- and T2-weighted images, and demonstrate diffuse heterogeneous enhancement.
▶ Littoral cell angioma: vascular benign splenic tumor typically hypointense on T2-weighted images.

Teaching Points

Although splenic hemangiomata are rare, they are the most common primary tumor of the spleen. They are usually asymptomatic but may cause abdominal discomfort when large. Diffuse hemangiomatosis of the spleen is a rare manifestation of systemic angiomatosis (Klippel-Trenaunay-Weber, Beckwith-Wiedemann syndromes). There may be an associated coagulopathy. Rare cases of malignant degeneration have been reported.

Splenic hemangiomas consist of the same proliferation of abnormal vascular channels as hepatic hemangiomas and thus can have similar appearances on imaging: hyperintense on T2-weighted images, and hypointense on T1-weighted images. However, there can be variable amounts of hemosiderin deposition leading to decreased signal intensity on both T1- and T2-weighted images. Progressive centripetal enhancement with persistent uniform enhancement on delayed imaging is characteristic although not frequently seen. Other patterns of enhancement are more frequently seen and include centripetal enhancement from the periphery, which persists on delayed images, early diffuse hyperenhancement, or mottled enhancement with foci of fibrosis or cysts (seen in one-third of cases) which remain hypoenhancing relative to spleen. When the appearance is equivocal, a Tc-99m labeled red cell scan may confirm the diagnosis by demonstrating increased activity on delayed images.

Management

Splenic hemangiomas grow slowly over time and may become symptomatic in adulthood. Large lesions may cause spontaneous splenic rupture requiring emergency surgery.

Further Readings

1. Vilanova JC, Barcelo J, et al. Hemangioma from head to toe: MR imaging with pathologic correlation. *RadioGraphics*. 2004; *24*(2): 367–385.
2. Elsayes KM, Narra VR, et al. MR imaging of the spleen: spectrum of abnormalities. *RadioGraphics*. 2005; *25*(4): 967–982.

History

▶ 48-year-old man with incidentally detected splenic mass on CT.

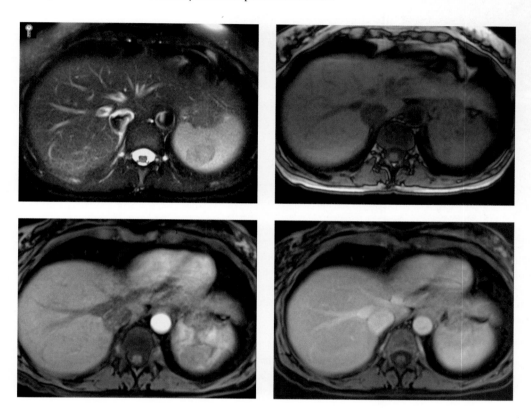

Case 155 Splenic Hamartoma

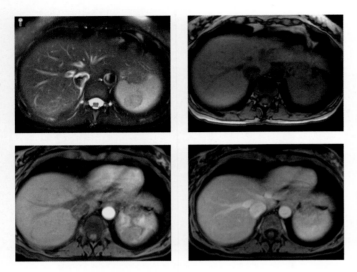

Findings

Fat-suppressed T2-weighted (top right), T1-weighted (top left), and gadolinium-enhanced arterial phase (bottom right) and portal venous phase (bottom left) MR images show a well circumscribed 4 cm isolated splenic mass. The lesion is isointense to splenic parenchyma on T1 and heterogeneously mildly hypointense on T2. There is mild, early heterogeneous enhancement during the arterial phase and uniform enhancement on the delayed phase of contrast enhancement.

Differential Diagnosis

▶ Hemangioma: most common primary benign splenic neoplasm. The majority of lesions are T1 hypointense, T2 hyperintense, and have early mottled enhancement with delayed hyperenhancement.

▶ Lymphoma: most common malignant splenic neoplasm. Often demonstrates T1 and T2 isointensity and homogeneous hypointense enhancement relative to normal spleen on post-gadolinium images.

▶ Splenic metastasis: relatively uncommon, particularly in the absence of widespread metastatic disease. Splenic metastases have a variable appearances depending on origin of the primary tumor.

Teaching Points

Splenic hamartomas are benign and usually asymptomatic lesions composed of an anomalous mixture of splenic red pulp. The incidence of splenic hamartomas ranges from 0.02 percent to 0.13 percent. On CT, hamartomas are often occult because they are isoattenuating prior to and following the administration of intravenous contrast. On MRI, the majority of hamartomas show heterogeneous hyperintensity relative to spleen on T2, diffuse early arterial enhancement, along with uniform and intense delayed enhancement following the administration of gadolinium. MRI is the diagnostic modality of choice for characterization.

Management

Although the radiologic features of splenic hamartomas may be suggestive, a definitive preoperative diagnosis is rarely made based on the imaging appearance alone. Surveillance with follow-up imaging to ensure stability as well as surgical resection has both been reported.

Further Readings

1. Elsayed KM, Narra VR, Makundan G et al. MR Imaging of the Spleen: Spectrum of Abnormalities. *RadioGraphics,* 2005; *25:* 967–982.
2. Abbott RM, Levy AD, Aguilera NS, et al. From the Archives of the AFIP Primary Vascular Neoplasms of the Spleen: Radiologic-Pathologic Correlation. *RadioGraphics.* 2004; *24:* 1137–1163.

History

▶ 69-year-old man with left upper quadrant pain.

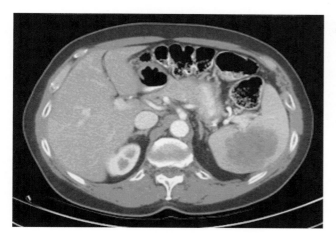

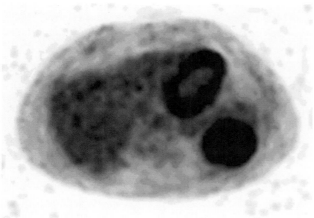

Case 156 Splenic Lymphoma

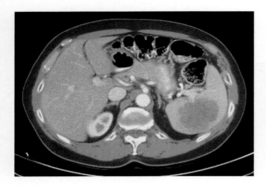 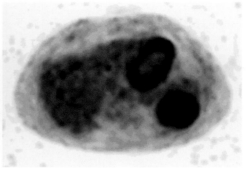

Findings

CT (left) shows a well-defined, round hypoattenuating splenic mass. PET-CT (right) shows a focal increased uptake within the spleen with a maximum SUV of 11.8. At surgery, a bulging tumor extending from the spleen into the adjacent diaphragm was found; pathology identified this lesion as diffuse large B-cell lymphoma.

Differential Diagnosis

► Hemangioma: have variable CT features; they may have marked homogeneous contrast enhancement, heterogeneous mottled enhancement, or peripheral enhancement with centripetal progression of contrast. In general, they do not have increased 18F-FDG uptake on PET-CT.

► Hamartoma: most often isoattenuating relative to normal spleen on intravenous contrast-enhanced CT. The most characteristic feature is hypervascularity on color Doppler sonography. They are not expected to show increased 18F-FDG uptake.

► Metastasis: have variable CT appearances and should always be considered in the differential of a solid splenic mass. Observing a primary malignancy on the scan or additional metastatic lesions can help suggest the diagnosis.

Teaching Points

Lymphomas are the most common primary splenic malignancy. Unlike incidentally discovered hemangiomas and hamartomas, patients with splenic lymphoma usually have symptoms such as left upper quadrant pain, fullness, or a palpable mass. Secondary splenic involvement is common in both non-Hodgkin (NHL) and Hodgkin lymphoma (HL); less commonly, the spleen is the primary organ of involvement. Primary low-grade NHL generally presents with relatively subtle parenchymal changes on CT or a hypoattenuating mass. Splenic involvement by aggressive high-grade NHL may present on CT as a large (frequently up to several centimeters in size) hypodense parenchymal mass with areas of necrosis and invasion into adjacent structures. Hodgkin lymphoma has an appearance intermediate to that of low- and high-grade NHL. FDG-PET/CT is reported to have an accuracy of almost 100 percent in diagnosing primary splenic involvement, while CT alone has a lower overall accuracy of approximately 57 percent.

Management

Patients with localized diffuse large B-cell lymphoma are generally treated with chemotherapy with or without radiotherapy.

Further Reading

1. Chua SC, Rozalli FI, O'Connor SR. Imaging features of primary extranodal lymphomas. *Clin Radiol.* 2009; 64: 574–588.

History

► 60-year-old female with a skin lesion.

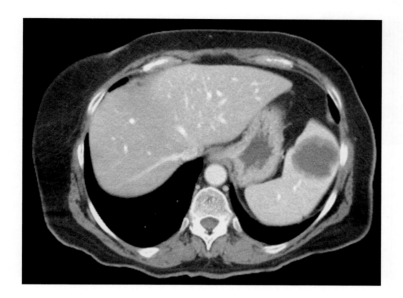

Case 157 Splenic Metastasis from Malignant Melanoma

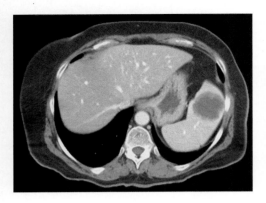

Findings

Axial contrast-enhanced CT shows a hypoattenuating mass with irregular borders and central necrosis located in the anterior aspect of the spleen.

Differential Diagnosis

▶ Abscess: may contain gas or dependent layering debris. Symptoms or signs of infection are typically present.

▶ Infarct: wedge-shaped and peripherally located.

▶ Hemangioma: appearance varies from solid to multicystic. Hemangiomas are usually hypodense without contrast and show delayed enhancement on contrast phases.

Teaching Points

Splenic metastasis is uncommon and occurs in a minority of patients with systemic metastatic disease. The most common route of spread is hematogenous, which occurs in breast cancer, lung cancer, and melanoma. Other routes of spread to the spleen include peritoneal implants to the capsule, most often from ovarian cancer, and direct invasion of tumors from surrounding organs. Solitary splenic metastasis in the absence of metastatic disease is occasionally seen with colorectal and ovarian carcinomas, often with a latency of several years after diagnosis of the primary tumor. Comparison with prior imaging to assess for interval growth or PET scans can be obtained to differentiate metastases from benign entities such as the more common hemangiomas and cysts. Percutaneous diagnostic biopsy should be obtained with caution owing to a concern for causing substantial hemorrhage.

Management

Management of splenic metastasis varies based on clinical setting, type of primary malignancy and extent of metastatic disease. Metastasis to the spleen in the absence of other metastatic disease is unusual. In most cases therapy is driven by management of extra-splenic metastatic disease.

Further Readings

1. Freeman JL, Jafri SZ, Roberts JL, Mezwa DG, Shirkhoda A. CT of congenital and acquired abnormalities of the spleen. *RadioGraphics*. 1993; *13*: 597–610.
2. Rabushka LS, Kawashima A, Fishman EK. Imaging of the spleen: CT with supplemental MR examination. *RadioGraphics*. 1994; *14*: 307–332.

History

▶ 40-year-old man, injured in a motor vehicle accident.

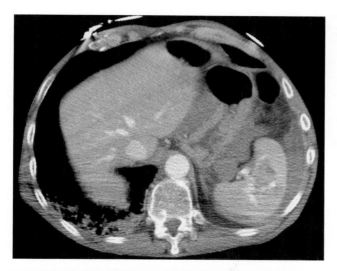

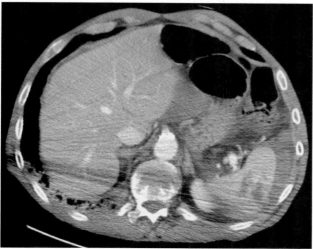

Case 158 Splenic Trauma

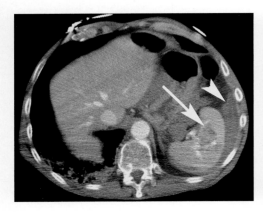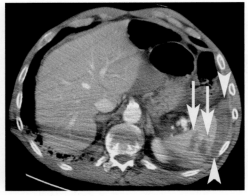

Findings

Contrast-enhanced CT images demonstrate multiple low-density deep linear lacerations in the mid spleen (arrows), extending from the lateral aspect to near the splenic hilum with moderate perisplenic hemoperitoneum (arrowheads). No definite active extravasation is seen.

Differential Diagnosis

▶ Splenic infarct: wedge-shaped area of low attenuation. No history of trauma, no hemoperitoneum.
▶ Splenic cyst or abscess: signs of infection are usually present with splenic abscess.
▶ Splenic cleft: variant in contour of spleen, no surrounding hemorrhage.

Teaching Points

The spleen is the most common organ injured in the setting of trauma requiring surgery. Patients may have left upper quadrant pain and hypotension. Traumatic injury can range from subcapsular hematomas to splenic lacerations and splenic fractures. A subcapsular hematoma typically compresses and flattens the lateral margin of the spleen. A laceration is a jagged linear area of nonenhancement. A splenic fracture is a deep laceration extending from outer capsule through splenic hilum. Secondary CT findings include hemoperitoneum or perisplenic clot which usually measures greater than 45 Hounsfield Units. In general, the highest attenuation extra-lumenal fluid in the abdomen is usually close in proximity to the site of bleeding (sentinel clot sign). Active arterial extravasation appears as an area of high-attenuation contrast material within a low-density hematoma.

Management

While the decision for surgery depends on clinical factors, CT helps diagnose and monitor the extent of injuries. Conservative measures are appropriate in the stable patient, but minor injuries can progress to delayed bleeding or rupture which may require embolization, splenectomy or splenorrhaphy.

Further Reading

1. Shanmugananthan K, Mirvis SE, Boyd-Kranis R, Takada T, Scalea TM. Nonsurgical management of blunt splenic injury: use of CT criteria to select patients for splenic arteriography and potential endovascular therapy. *Radiology*. 2000; *217*(1):75–82.

Part 12   **Mesentery and Peritoneum**

History

▶ 24-year-old woman complains of a 10-day history of increasing abdominal pain, weight loss, and fever.

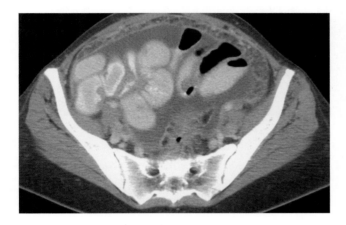

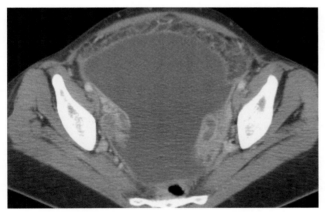

Case 159 Peritoneal Tuberculosis

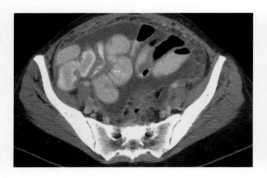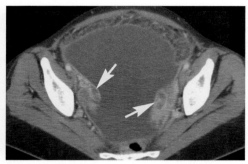

Findings

CT scans of the pelvis show a large amount of ascites, smoothly enhancing peritoneum, and innumerable enhancing nodules in the greater omentum. There are rim-enhancing, low-attenuation lymph nodes in the pelvis (arrows).

Differential Diagnosis

- ▶ Peritoneal carcinomatosis: nodular peritoneal implants with irregular thickening and enhancement suggest carcinomatosis. A smooth peritoneum with minimal thickening and pronounced enhancement suggests tuberculosis.
- ▶ Peritoneal lymphomatosis: lymph node enlargement in lymph node chains commonly involved with lymphoma suggests lymphoma.

Teaching Points

Mycobacterium tuberculosis reaches the peritoneal cavity as part of a systemic infection (miliary tuberculosis), direct extension from the bowel to the peritoneum, or lymphatic dissemination. It is an uncommon complication of tuberculosis infection in developed countries, where it occurs most commonly in immunocompromised patients. The volume of ascites in peritoneal tuberculosis is variable. Ascitic fluid may be diffuse or loculated and typically has higher attenuation than simple fluid. Enhancing soft tissue nodules usually stud the peritoneal surfaces and omentum and mesenteries. Peritoneal enhancement may occur and is usually smooth, in contrast to nodular enhancement that is more characteristic of peritoneal carcinomatosis. Lymph node enlargement in the peripancreatic and periportal regions, mesenteries, and retroperitoneum may also be present. It is not uncommon for tuberculous lymph nodes to have central low attenuation from caseous necrosis. Other findings in the abdomen, such as miliary microabscesses in the liver and/or spleen, splenomegaly, splenic or lymph node calcification, and inflammatory thickening of the terminal ileum and cecum, may help suggest tuberculosis as the etiology of diffuse peritoneal disease.

Management

For diagnostically ambiguous cases, minimally invasive procedures such as laparoscopic, endoscopic, and percutaneous biopsy can establish the case of peritoneal disease. Medical therapy is the mainstay of treatment. Surgical procedures are reserved for treatment of complications.

Further Readings

1. Ha HK, Jung JI, Lee MS, et al. CT differentiation of tuberculous peritonitis and peritoneal carcinomatosis. *Am J Roentgenol.* 1996;*167*(3):743–748.
2. Levy AD, Shaw JC, Sobin LH. Secondary tumors and tumorlike lesions of the peritoneal cavity: imaging features with pathologic correlation. *RadioGraphics.* 2009;*29*(2):347–373.

History

▶ 77-year-old woman with abdominal distention and pain.

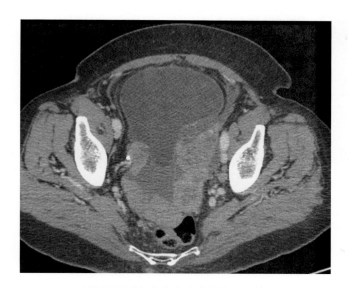

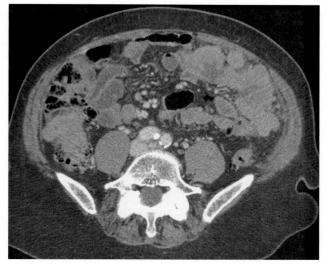

Case 160 Peritoneal Carcinomatosis

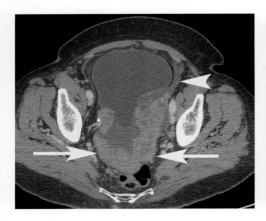
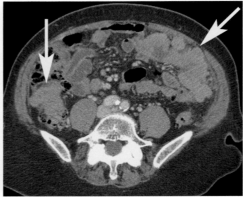

Findings

Axial CT image (left) through the pelvis shows ascites (arrowhead) and extensive soft tissue masses (arrows) within the cul-de-sac. More cephalad axial image (right) demonstrates additional, large, peritoneal soft-tissue masses (arrows).

Differential Diagnosis

▶ Peritoneal lymphomatosis: may be indistinguishable from carcinomatosis, but often has mesenteric lymphadenopathy and splenomegaly.
▶ Primary peritoneal mesothelioma: patients may have prior asbestos exposure.
▶ Peritoneal tuberculosis: peritoneal masses are typically smoother than in carcinomatosis and may be associated with low density lymphadenopathy and history of TB exposure.

Teaching Points

Peritoneal carcinomatosis is the spread of cancer cells along the peritoneal lining, usually associated with ovarian and gastrointestinal tract adenocarcinomas. The most common sites for peritoneal implants are those where flow of fluid is arrested such as the cul-de-sac, right paracolic gutter, Morrison pouch (also called Morison pouch) and surrounding the sigmoid colon. Other common sites of implants are the right hemidiaphragm, liver and omentum. CT findings include solitary or multiple peritoneal soft tissue masses (implants), irregular omental soft tissue plaques (omental cake) and ascites. Sheets of tumor cells may present as linear thickening and enhancement of the peritoneal surfaces. Serosal implants may cause small bowel tethering or bowel obstruction.

Management

Peritoneal carcinomatosis is a poor prognostic finding. Mainstays of treatment are surgical cytoreduction (particularly in ovarian carcinoma) and platinum or taxane-based chemotherapy. Neoadjuvant chemotherapy, followed by surgical debulking, has been shown to improve outcomes in select patients. Contrast-enhanced CT and FDG-PET (usually with combined modality CT) are complementary in disease monitoring and response to therapy, though each has sensitivity limitations. Tumor markers, such as CA-125 in ovarian carcinoma, are also commonly used to monitor disease progression and response to therapy.

Further Readings

1. Smiti S, Rajagopal K. CT mimics of peritoneal carcinomatosis. *Indian J Radiol Imaging.* 2010; *20*(1):58–62.
2. Pannu HK, Bristow RE, Montz FJ, Fishman EK. Multidetector CT of peritoneal carcinomatosis from ovarian cancer. *RadioGraphics.* 2003; *23*:687–701.

History

▶ 55-year-old man who worked in a shipyard complained of abdominal discomfort and fullness.

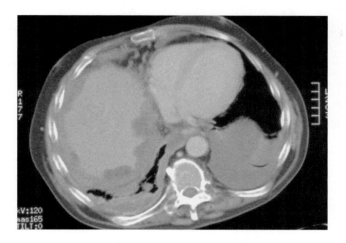

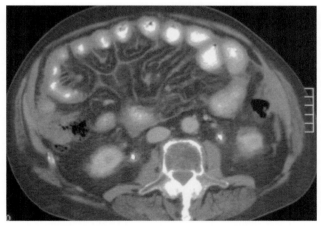

Case 161 Malignant Mesothelioma

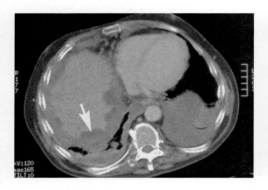 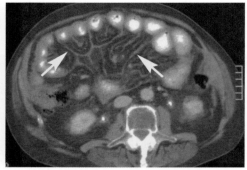

Findings

CT shows complex ascites and peritoneal implants that scallop the liver margin (arrow on left image) as well as a left pleural effusion and nodular thickening of the right pleura. There is pleating of the mesentery (arrows on right image) and thickening of the small bowel wall.

Differential Diagnosis

► Peritoneal carcinomatosis: more common than and usually indistinguishable from malignant mesothelioma. Other findings suggesting malignant mesothelioma include lack of significant lymphadenopathy, evidence of asbestos exposure, and absence of a primary malignancy.

► Peritoneal lymphomatosis: secondary involvement of the peritoneum from nodal or extranodal lymphomas may appear identical to malignant mesothelioma and peritoneal carcinomatosis. The presence of adenopathy in lymph node chains typically involved with lymphoma such as the small bowel mesentery or retrocrural region suggests lymphoma.

► Tuberculous peritonitis: peritoneal tuberculosis may have omental nodules but does not usually produce peritoneal masses. Low attenuation lymphadenopathy, ileocecal inflammatory disease, and miliary disease in the liver or spleen suggest tuberculosis.

Teaching Points

Malignant mesothelioma is an uncommon, aggressive malignant neoplasm that arises from mesothelial cells. It has a strong association with asbestos exposure. The majority of malignant mesotheliomas arise from the pleura. Peritoneal primaries account for 6 to 10 percent of malignant mesotheliomas. Peritoneal malignant mesothelioma may diffusely involve the peritoneum or may be localized, presenting as a solitary mass. The diffuse form is characterized by tumor infiltrating and thickening the peritoneum in a sheet-like fashion. Omental caking, ascites, and infiltration of the small bowel mesentery are usually present. The small bowel mesentery may have pleated or stellate pattern on imaging. Localized peritoneal malignant mesothelioma is a heterogeneous, solid intraperitoneal mass with irregular margins. Invasion of adjacent visceral structures such as the liver, spleen, or pelvic organs may occur.

Management

Diffuse malignant mesotheliomas are highly aggressive and with few exceptions are incurable. Patients with localized malignant mesotheliomas usually have a good prognosis following complete surgical excision.

Further Reading

1. Levy AD, Arnaiz J, Shaw JC, Sobin LH. From the archives of the AFIP: primary peritoneal tumors: imaging features with pathologic correlation. *RadioGraphics*. 2008; *28*(2):583–607.

History

▶ 27-year-old woman with history of appendectomy, now with lower abdominal pain.

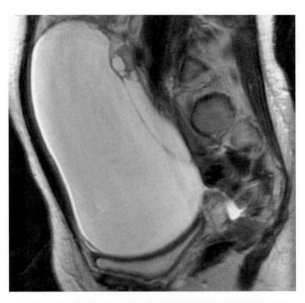

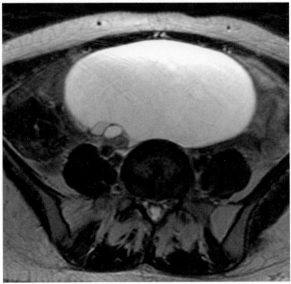

Case 162 Peritoneal Inclusion Cyst

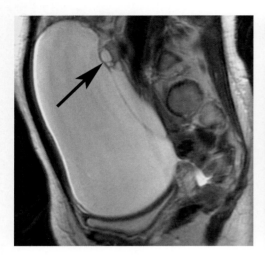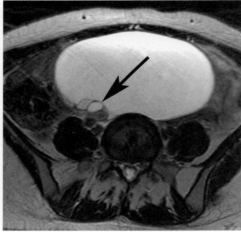

Findings

T2-weighted MR images in the coronal (left image) and axial (right image) plane show a large septated cyst with high T2 signal. The cyst surrounds the right ovary (arrow).

Differential Diagnosis

► Ovarian cyst: arises within the ovary: a "claw sign"—ovarian tissue surrounding a portion of a large cyst—suggests that the cyst originates in the ovary.
► Paraovarian cyst: a cyst within the broad ligament that is distinguished from peritoneal inclusion cyst by location adjacent to, but not surrounding, an ovary.
► Lymphocele: postoperative collection of lymphatic fluid, often located along the pelvic sidewalls but not typically surrounding an ovary.

Teaching Points

Peritoneal inclusion cysts occur exclusively in premenopausal women. Normal ovaries release physiologic fluid into the peritoneal space. Peritoneal inclusion cysts are due to periadnexal adhesions, such as may occur after pelvic inflammatory disease or surgery, resulting in loculated accumulation of released fluid around the ovary. These benign collections may cause pain due to mass effect. Imaging is useful in establishing this diagnosis by determining the relationship of the fluid collection to the ovary. Cysts may occasionally be hemorrhagic and show high attenuation on CT and high signal on T1 and low signal on T2 weighted imaging. Peritoneal inclusion cysts have been referred to as benign multicystic mesotheliomas, but this terminology is now generally felt to be incorrect as the mesothelial cells lining the inclusion cyst have no pathologic similarity to those of malignant mesothelioma.

Management

Oral contraceptives may reduce the volume of ovarian fluid associated with ovulation. Symptomatic cysts may require surgery; recurrence is frequent.

Further Readings

1. Moyle PL, Kataoka MY, Nakai A, Takahata A, Reinhold C, Sala E. Nonovarian cystic lesions of the pelvis. *RadioGraphics.* 2010; *30*:921–938.
2. Chang WC, Meux MD, Yeh BM, Qayyum A, Joe BN, Chen LM, Coakley FV. CT and MRI of adnexal masses in patients with primary nonovarian malignancy. *Am J Roentgenol.* 2006; *186*(4):1039–1045.

History

▶ 33-year-old man complains of increasing abdominal girth and abdominal pain.

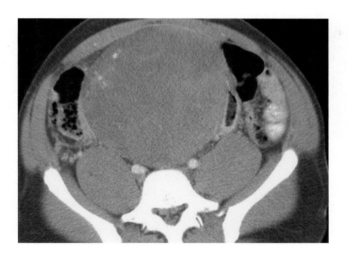

Case 163 Mesenteric Fibromatosis

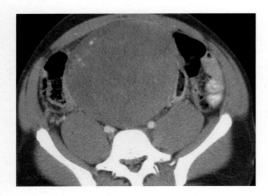

Findings

Large, heterogeneous, low-attenuation soft tissue mass in the mid abdomen, most likely arising from the small bowel mesentery. There is mass effect on the adjacent bowel.

Differential Diagnosis

▶ Lymphoma: lymph node enlargement in adjacent lymph node chains or elsewhere in the body suggests lymphoma.

▶ Metastatic disease: multifocality, ascites, peritoneal thickening, and disease in other organs suggest metastatic disease.

▶ Soft tissue sarcoma: may occur in the mesentery, but is more common in the retroperitoneum and extremities.

▶ Gastrointestinal stromal tumors (GIST): small bowel GISTs may have an extensive mesenteric component or may occur primarily in the mesentery. Large GISTs typically contain areas of hemorrhage and necrosis, manifesting as focal areas of hypoattenuation.

Teaching Points

Mesenteric fibromatosis, also called intraabdominal fibromatosis or abdominal desmoid, is a benign fibroproliferative process that is locally aggressive and has the capacity to recur following resection. It occurs throughout a wide age range (14 to 75 years, mean 41 years) and does not have a gender predilection. Although most cases occur sporadically, 13 percent of patients have familial adenomatous polyposis. Histologically, lesions may have a collagenous or myxoid stroma, or both. Collagenous portions are typically homogeneous, soft tissue attenuation on CT, and myxoid stroma is hypoattenuating. Lesions with both myxoid and collagenous stroma may have a striated or whorled appearance due to alternating collagenous and myxoid areas. Intravenous contrast enhancement patterns vary, from mild homogeneous enhancement to heterogeneous enhancement. Predominantly myxoid lesions typically remain hypoattenuating and do not enhance with intravenous contrast enhancement. On MR, myxoid stromal elements contribute to high signal intensity on T2-weighted images

Management

Following resection, local recurrence is common and primary disease in the bowel mesentery may be complicated by small bowel obstruction and fistula formation. Some authors recommend wide surgical excision, while others recommend less radical surgery or medical therapy with antiestrogens or cytotoxic chemotherapy.

Further Reading

1. Levy AD, Rimola J, Mehrotra AK, Sobin LH. From the archives of the AFIP: benign fibrous tumors and tumorlike lesions of the mesentery: radiologic-pathologic correlation. *RadioGraphics*. 2006; 26(1):245–264.

History

▶ 80-year-old man complains of abdominal pain.

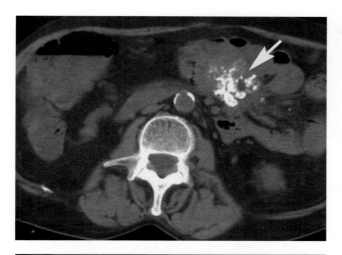

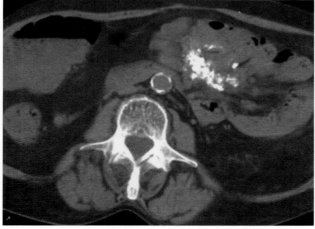

Case 164 Sclerosing Mesenteritis

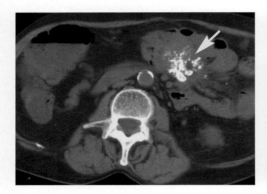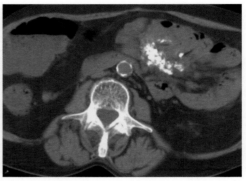

Findings

Enhanced CT shows a soft tissue attenuation mesenteric mass that contains dense central calcifications (arrow). The mass is adherent to adjacent small bowel. There is no associated bowel dilatation or obstruction.

Differential Diagnosis

▸ Metastasis: mucinous adenocarcinoma, mucinous ovarian cancer, and carcinoid metastasis may contain calcification.
▸ Lymphoma: following treatment lymphoma may calcify.

Teaching Points

Sclerosing mesenteritis is also known as mesenteric panniculitis, retractile mesenteritis and mesenteric lipodystrophy. It is an idiopathic disorder that produces haziness, soft-tissue infiltration, or tumor-like masses within the mesentery. Histologically, it is characterized by chronic, nonspecific inflammation, fat necrosis, and fibrosis. It usually occurs in middle-aged men. and the most common symptom is abdominal pain. The small bowel mesentery is the most common location. It may also arise in the transverse mesocolon and omenta. Initially, there is nonspecific inflammation within the mesentery that may progress to fat necrosis and fibrosis. The mesentery can become thickened and shortened, which may result in kinking or fixation of the adjacent bowel. There is a tendency for the process to preserve normal fat around the vessels or aggregates of lymphoid cells, which is known as the "fat ring sign" or "halo sign" when observed on CT.

Management

Sclerosing mesenteritis is often self-limiting. The treatment is controversial. Some authors recommend close clinical observation while others treat with prednisone and azathioprine. Surgical treatment is usually reserved for patients that have complications such as small bowel obstruction or perforation.

Further Readings

1. Levy AD, Rimola J, Mehrotra AK, Sobin LH. From the archives of the AFIP: benign fibrous tumors and tumorlike lesions of the mesentery: radiologic-pathologic correlation. *RadioGraphics*. 2006; *26*(1):245–264.
2. Horton KM, Lawler LP, Fishman EK. CT findings in sclerosing mesenteritis (panniculitis): spectrum of disease. *RadioGraphics*. 2003; *23*(6):1561–1567.

History

▶ 21-year-old woman complains of vague right upper quadrant pain.

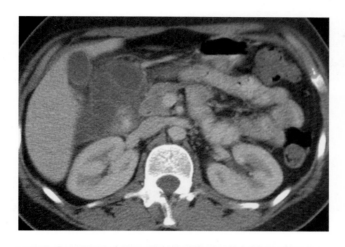

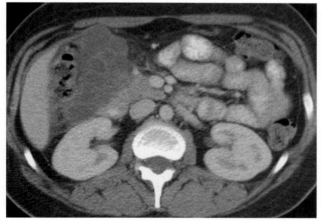

Case 165 Lymphangioma

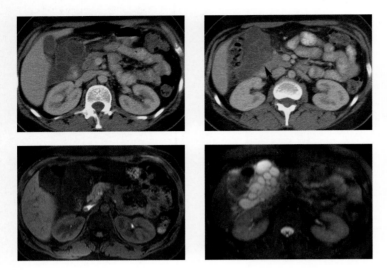

Findings

There is a multilocular cystic mass adjacent to the head of the pancreas. The mass abuts the hepatic flexure of the colon. Additional T1- and T2-weighted MR images at the same level signal intensity within the cystic mass that is consistent with simple fluid.

Differential Diagnosis

- ▶ Pancreatic pseudocyst: tends to be unilocular, but may appear more complicated when there is secondary infection or hemorrhage. Typically, the patient has a clinical history of pancreatitis.
- ▶ Pancreatic microcystic serous adenoma: multiloculated cystic mass that arises from the pancreas and is composed of numerous small cysts and thin septations, which coalesce centrally to from a scar. Central calcification may be present.
- ▶ Enteric duplication cyst: unilocular or multilocular cystic lesion that is most often associated with the bowel. Occasionally, it may be located a distance from the bowel within a supporting mesentery.

Teaching Points

Lymphangiomas are benign lesions composed of thin-walled cystic spaces and lymphatic-like vessels. The majority (95 percent) of lymphangiomas are located in the head and neck region. The abdomen is the second most common location, accounting for 5 percent of lesions. On imaging, they are unilocular or multilocular fluid-attenuation masses. Rarely, the cyst fluid has negative attenuation values indicating the presence of chyle. Hemorrhage and infection may complicate lymphangiomas and alter the attenuation or signal intensity of the cyst fluid. The cyst walls and septa enhance after intravenous contrast administration. Abdominal lymphangiomas may be located in the mesentery or retroperitoneum or associated with the intestine. Rarely, they may occur in the liver, gallbladder, spleen, pancreas, or kidney.

Management

Surgical resection is generally indicated to establish the diagnosis and relieve symptoms of mass effect on adjacent organs or vasculature.

Further Readings

1. Zhu H, Wu ZY, Lin XZ, Shi B, Upadhyaya M, Chen K. Gastrointestinal tract lymphangiomas: findings at CT and endoscopic imaging with histopathologic correlation. *Abdom Imaging*. 2008; *33*(6):662–668.
2. Levy AD, Cantisani V, Miettinen M. Abdominal lymphangiomas: imaging features with pathologic correlation. *Am J Roentgenol*.2004; *182*(6):1485–1491.

History

▶ 40-year-old man complains of abdominal pain following a motor vehicle accident.

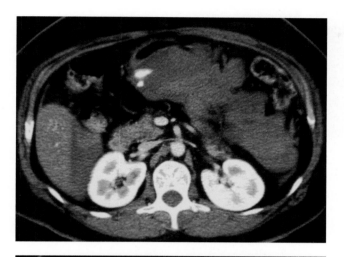

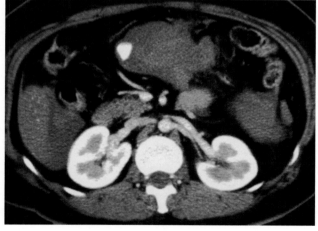

Case 166 Mesenteric Hematoma

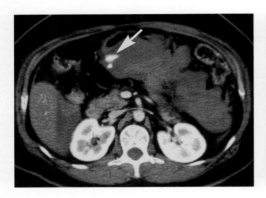
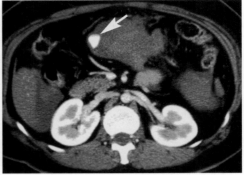

Findings

A large heterogeneous mass with central high attenuation involves the transverse mesocolon. Active extravasation of intravenous contrast (arrows) indicates active hemorrhage. The adjacent bowel is normal in appearance.

Differential Diagnosis

► Mesenteric bleeding: suggested in the setting of blunt abdominal trauma, high attenuation fluid and active extravasation within a mesentery. If the CT scan had been performed with bowel contrast, a bowel perforation would have been a possibility; free air would most likely be present.

Teaching Points

Mesenteric hemorrhage in the setting of blunt trauma is uncommon. When detected, reporting the severity of the hemorrhage and the presence or absence of significant bowel injury (laceration, perforation, or ischemia) is critical to triage patients to surgical intervention or observation. Mesenteric hematomas tend to be focal, well-defined masses that are the result of mesenteric vascular laceration. They may be triangular, round, or oval in shape. Acute hemorrhage is generally high in attenuation (50 to 60 HU) and becomes less attenuating over time. The finding of intravenous contrast extravasation in the region of the hematoma is indicative of active bleeding. Irregularity of the mesenteric vessels, often termed mesenteric beading, and abrupt termination of vessels may also indicate mesenteric vascular injury. In some cases, the hemorrhage in the mesentery is less well defined such that the mesentery appears hazy, infiltrated, or indistinct.

Management

The finding of active hemorrhage within a mesenteric hematoma or associated bowel perforation or ischemia indicates surgery is necessary. Less significant injuries such as an isolated mesenteric hematoma without evidence of active bleeding can be managed conservatively.

Further Readings

1. Dowe, M. F., Shanmuganathan, K., Mirvis, S. E., Steiner, R. C. and Cooper, C . CT findings of mesenteric injury after blunt trauma: implications for surgical intervention. *Am J Roentgenol.* 1997; *168*:425–428.
2. Hanks, P. W. and Brody, J. M . Blunt injury to mesentery and small bowel: CT evaluation. *Radiol Clin North Am.* 2003; *41*:1171–1182.

History

▶ 53-year-old woman who recently underwent bariatric surgery presents with acute abdominal pain.

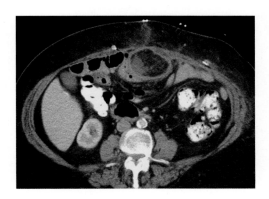

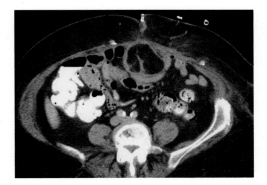

Case 167   Omental Infarction

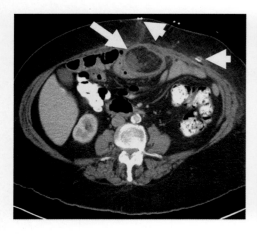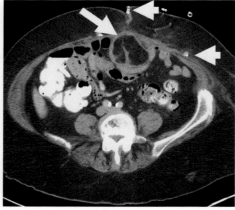

Findings

CT images show a mixed attenuation, predominantly fatty, intraperitoneal mass (long arrow) adjacent to the anterior abdominal wall. The mass displaces adjacent small bowel loops. Skin staples and a surgical drain are present (short arrows).

Differential Diagnosis

▶ Epiploic appendagitis: similar to omental infarction in both symptomatology and imaging appearance. May be distinguished by its smaller size and characteristic location adjacent to the colon.

▶ Mesenteric panniculitis: idiopathic inflammation in the mesenteric fat that manifests as hazy infiltrative stranding, nodular sub-centimeter lymphoid aggregates, venous engorgement, and frequently a thin hyperattenuating anterior rim. The infiltrative stranding spares the vessels and lymphoid aggregates. Often an incidental finding.

▶ Liposarcoma: may have an appearance similar to omental infarction but the patient should lack a history of acute onset abdominal pain.

Teaching Points

Infarction of the greater omentum typically presents with acute onset abdominal pain, possibly accompanied by nausea and/or vomiting. Male and obese patients are at greatest risk. Infarction occurs secondary to venous occlusion from etiologies such as omental torsion, adhesions, or prior surgery. On imaging, omental infarction presents as a large, heterogeneous and ill-defined fatty mass in the anterior abdomen typically remote from the colon and most commonly occurs in the right lower quadrant.

Management

Omental infarcts may be treated nonsurgically with nonsteroidal anti-inflammatory medications for symptomatic relief.

Further Readings

1. Singh AK, Gervais DA, Lee S, et al. Omental infarct: CT imaging features. *Abdominal Imaging.* 2006; *31*(5): 549–554.
2. Singh AK, Gervais DA, Hahn PF, et al. Acute epiploic appendagitis and its mimics. *RadioGraphics.* 2005; *25*(6): 1521–1534.

History

▶ 87-year-old man with a left lateral abdominal mass/protrusion for approximately nine months.

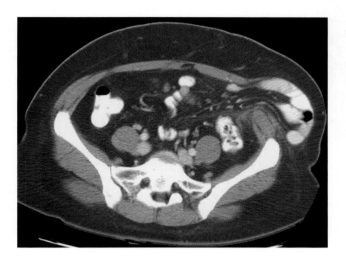

Case 168 Spigelian Hernia

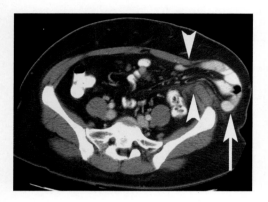

Findings

Transverse contrast-enhanced CT through the pelvis shows protrusion of fat and bowel (arrow) through an anterior abdominal wall defect (arrowheads) between the rectus abdominis and lateral abdominal wall muscles.

Differential Diagnosis

► Ventral hernia: herniation through midline fascial layers of the anterior abdominal wall.
► Parastomal hernia: herniation through a defect caused by colostomy or ileostomy placement.

Teaching Points

Spigelian hernias involve protrusion of omental fat, bowel, or other intra-abdominal contents through a defect in the Spigelian aponeurosis, located along the lateral margin of the rectus abdominis muscle at the semi-lunar line. This type of hernia has become more common as laparoscopic port sites are often placed in this location. They most commonly occur in middle-aged adults, but can present at any age, including in children. A Spigelian hernia may present as an incidental, asymptomatic finding, with slight swelling or localized pain, or as a frank bowel obstruction. The abdominal contents may protrude into the subcutaneous fat, but commonly dissect between the internal and external oblique muscles. It is important in cases of bowel obstruction to look for associated signs of bowel strangulation (i.e. circumferentially thickened bowel wall, pneumatosis intestinalis, free fluid, or absent or decreased bowel wall enhancement).

Management

Since Spigelian hernias are prone to obstruction and strangulation, they are optimally managed surgically. Smaller defects may be more prone to such complications, and some larger defects may be managed more conservatively. Surgical repair can be performed with open or laparoscopic techniques, and larger defects typically require mesh placement. Recurrence is rare, as most defects are small.

Further Readings

1. Aguirre DA, Casola G, Sirlin C. Abdominal Wall Hernias: MDCT findings. *Am J Roentgenol.* 2004; *183*(3):681–690.
2. Bittner JG, Edwards MA, Shah MB, MacFadyen BV, Mellinger JD. Mesh-free laparoscopic Spigelian hernia repair. *Am Surg.* 2008; *74*(8):713–720.
3. Furukawa A, Yamasaki M, Furuichi K, Yokoyama K, Nagata T, Takahashi M, Murata K, Sakamoto T. Helical CT in the Diagnosis of Small Bowel Obstruction. *RadioGraphics.* 2001; *21*:341–355.

History

► 53-year-old man complains of intermittent fevers for several months and slowly progressive right lower quadrant pain.

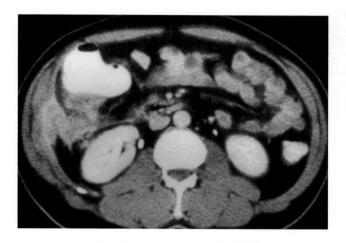

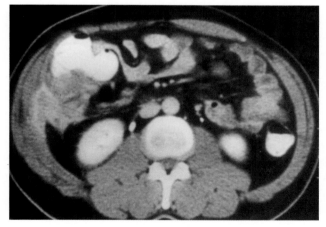

Case 169 Actinomycosis

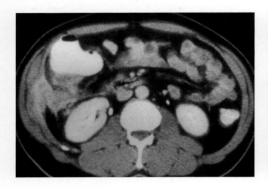 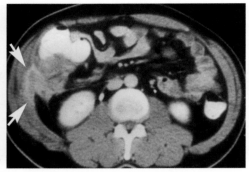

Findings

CT image show a heterogeneously enhancing mass that involves the posterior wall of the cecum and extends posteriorly into the percolonic fat, anterior limb of Gerota fascia, and into the right lateral abdominal wall musculature (arrows). The infiltration of the abdominal wall musculature has a peripheral rim of enhancement.

Differential Diagnosis

► Cecal adenocarcinoma: the asymmetric cecal wall thickening and extension into the abdominal wall is suggestive of an aggressive malignancy.
► Right-sided diverticulitis: is usually associated with acute inflammatory changes in the surrounding fat. The presence of diverticuli would also support the diagnosis.
► Crohn disease: the abscesses and fistulas in Crohn disease may involve the abdominal wall; however, in this case the terminal ileum is normal without other supportive features of Crohn disease.

Teaching Points

Actinomycosis is caused by *Actinomyces israelii*, a gram positive anaerobic bacteria, which is a normal human commensal organism in the oral cavity and gastrointestinal and genitourinary tracts. Although the pathogenesis of infection is not clearly understood, actinomyces may become invasive when mucosal barriers are disrupted from surgery, perforation, or trauma. Infection is most common in the head and neck, followed by the chest, and abdomen. In the abdomen, the ileocecal region is the most common location. Infection is characterized by a slowly progressive inflammatory process with multiple abscesses, sinus tracts, and fistulae. The inflammatory mass consists of granulation and fibrous tissue. Clinical observation of characteristic sulfur granules in the pus or drainage fluid on Papanicolaou smears suggests the diagnosis. Definitive diagnosis is by isolation of the bacteria in culture medium or histology.

Management

Treatment of actinomycosis requires long courses of penicillin or macrolides such as tetracycline or erythromycin. In some cases, surgery may be necessary.

Further Readings

1. Thanos L, Mylona S, Kalioras V, Pomoni M, Batakis N. Ileocecal actinomycosis: a case report. *Abdom Imaging.* 2004;29(1):36–38.
2. Yenarkarn P, Thoeni RF, Hanks D. Case 117: actinomycosis of left kidney with sinus tracts. *Radiology.* 2007;244(1):309–313.

History

▶ 17-year-old boy complains of right lower quadrant pain and fever.

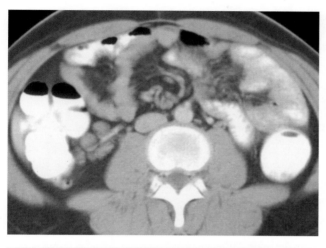

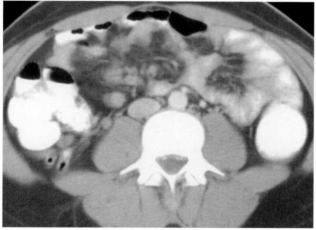

Case 170 Mesenteric Adenitis

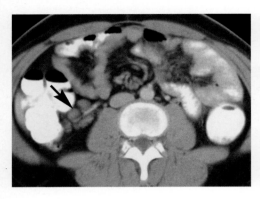
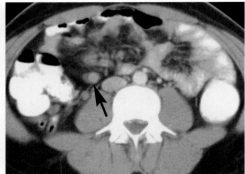

Findings

CT shows a cluster of homogeneously attenuating lymph nodes (arrows) in the right lower quadrant ileocecal mesentery. The appendix and cecum are normal.

Differential Diagnosis

▶ Normal lymph nodes: in children and adolescents, the finding of small lymph nodes in the small bowel mesentery is common.

▶ Secondary mesenteric lymphadenitis: mesenteric lymphadenitis occurring in the setting of a detectable or known inflammatory condition such as Crohn disease, ulcerative colitis, infectious ileitis or colitis, cecal diverticulitis, or HIV infection.

▶ Neoplastic lymph node enlargement: lymph node enlargement greater than 1 cm short axis, particularly in the setting of a known primary malignancy. However, size criteria are neither sensitive nor specific for predicting the presence of malignancy

Teaching Points

The diagnosis of mesenteric adenitis is made when there is a cluster of inflammatory lymph nodes in the right lower quadrant ileocecal mesentery in children, adolescents, and young adults in the clinical setting of right lower quadrant pain. It is an uncommon cause of right lower quadrant pain in adults. Mesenteric adenitis may be referred to as primary when there is no identifiable cause of inflammation in the right lower quadrant or as secondary when there is a detectable cause of inflammation such as appendicitis, diverticulitis, or inflammatory bowel disease. The lymph nodes in mesenteric adenitis are usually homogeneous in CT attenuation and less than 10 mm in diameter. In primary mesenteric adenitis, mild terminal ileal wall thickening (less than 5 mm) may be present.

Management

Mesenteric adenitis is treated conservatively. Endoscopy and further imaging may be performed in patients whose symptoms do not resolve to look for an underlying inflammatory or neoplastic etiology within the small bowel or colon.

Further Readings

1. Macari M, Hines J, Balthazar E, Megibow A. Mesenteric adenitis: CT diagnosis of primary versus secondary causes, incidence, and clinical significance in pediatric and adult patients. *Am J Roentgenol.* 2002; *178*(4):853–858.
2. Lucey BC, Stuhlfaut JW, Soto JA. Mesenteric lymph nodes seen at imaging: causes and significance. *RadioGraphics.* 2005; *25*(2):351–365.

History

▶ 58-year-old man with history of lung cancer.

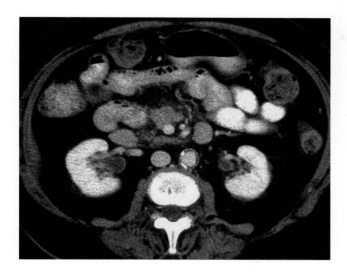

Case 171 Mesenteric Metastasis

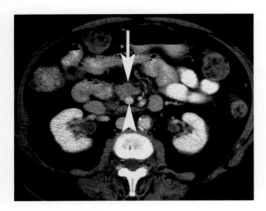

Findings

CT image shows soft tissue mass (arrow) that has broad contact with the superior mesenteric vein (arrowhead).

Differential Diagnosis

► Lymphoma: well-defined and typically homogeneous attenuation. Prominent lymphadenopathy is seen in most cases.

► Pancreatic adenocarcinoma: involves the pancreas.

► Sclerosing mesenteritis: associated with more extensive mesenteric fat stranding, and associated enlarged lymph aggregates may show local surrounding lower- attenuation fat.

Teaching Points

Mesenteric masses and metastases are commonly missed owing to their similarity in appearance to bowel. A helpful discriminator between bowel and mesenteric masses is that mesenteric veins and arteries greater than 1 mm in diameter are typically completely encased by a layer of fat. As such, the finding of an absent fat plane between what appears to be bowel and a mesenteric vessel should raise the concern that an underlying abnormality may be present. Further inspection of the images or reimaging may then help distinguish between bowel and a mass or inflammation in that region. Exceptions to this rule are the duodenum and the very proximal jejunum in the left upper abdomen, where mesenteric vessels do not have an intervening fat plane with bowel in normal individuals. The pancreatic head almost invariably shows contact with the superior mesenteric vein.

Management

Careful inspection of mesenteric vessels to identify areas with vascular contact with soft tissue assists in the detection of mesenteric abnormalities. Reimaging may be helpful in ambiguous cases.

Further Reading

1. Yeh BM, Joe BN, Sirlin CB, Webb EM, Westphalen AC, Qayyum A, Coakley FV. Vascular contact with soft tissue: a sign of mesenteric masses at computed tomography. *J Comput Assist Tomogr.* 2008; *32*(2):185–190.

Index of Cases

Index

hepatitis, 240
hepatitis B, 178
hepatitis C, 177, 178, 205, 223
hepatocellular
    adenoma, 176, 198, 200, 204, 208, 222
    carcinoma, 172, 178, 192, 198, 200, 202, 204, 206, 208, 214, 222, 223, 270
hepatoduodenal ligament lymph nodes, 226
hereditary hemochromatosis, 182
hereditary nonpolyposis colon carcinoma, 100
hernia
    Amyand's syndrome, 128
    Spigelian, 360
herpes esophagitis, 12
heterotopic pancreas, 60
hiatal hernia, 26, 28, 65
"hidebound bowel" sign, 118
hilar cholangiocarcinoma, 270
hilar liver metastasis, 270
Hirschsprung disease, 76
HIV. *See* human immunodeficiency virus (HIV) infection
Hodgkin lymphoma, 334
human immunodeficiency virus (HIV) infection, 11, 364
    AIDS cholangiopathy, 266
    colorectal lymphoma, 154
    esophagitis, 12
hydatid cysts, 228, 230, 232
hyperfunctioning endocrine tumor, pancreas, 304
hyperparathyroidism, 61
hypervascular liver metastasis, 172, 214
hypervascular metastases, 192, 196, 200, 218
hypopharynx, 32

iatrogenic perforation, 24
idiopathic hepatic steatosis, 174
ileal carcinoid, 96
ileal pouches, 100
ileocolic tuberculosis, 92
ileostomies, 100
ileus, 152
incarcerated inguinal hernia, 128
infarct, 336, 338
infarction, omental, 358
infectious
    colitis, 138, 140, 144, 146, 364
    enteritis, 86, 88
    ileitis, 364

proctitis, 154
rectal wall thickening, 158
infiltrating pancreatic carcinoma, 320
infiltrative pancreatic adenocarcinoma, 286
inflammatory bowel disease, 136, 140, 142, 146, 154, 160
    Crohn disease, 44
    primary sclerosing cholangitis, 264
inflammatory disease of terminal ileum, 162
inflammatory pseudopolyps, 160
    ulcerative colitis with, 136
inflammatory rectal wall thickening, 158
inflammatory wall thickening, 240
inguinal hernia, acute appendicitis in, 128
insulin dependent diabetes mellitus, 316
insulinoma, 40, 302, 310
intestinal obstruction, 316
intraabdominal fibromatosis, 350
intraductal papillary mucinous neoplasm (IPMN), 284, 290, 294
    combined-duct type, 298
    multiple, 318
    side branch, 292, 300
intraductal papillary mucinous tumor, 274
intrahepatic cholangiocarcinoma, 196, 202, 206, 216
    peripheral, 196, 210
intraluminal duodenal diverticulum, 76
intramural esophageal dissection, 14
intramural pseudodiverticulosis with reflux stricture, 14
intrapancreatic accessory spleen, 312
intussusception, 244
inverted Meckel diverticulum, 111
ischemia, 154
ischemic colitis, 108, 134, 140, 146
ischemic enteritis, 88
islet cell tumors of pancreas, 284

jaundice, 71, 179, 189, 269, 275
jejunal
    adenocarcinoma, 100
    diverticulitis, 100, 120
    diverticulosis, 118
juvenile polyposis, 48, 98
juxta-papillary diverticulum, 74

Killian-Jamieson diverticulum, 34
Killian triangle, 34
Klatskin tumor, 270
Klebsiella, 328